CHRONIC PAIN

SOCIOLOGICAL OBSERVATIONS

Series Editor: **JOHN M. JOHNSON**, *Arizona State University*

"This new series seeks its inspiration primarily from its subject matter and the nature of its observational setting. It draws on all academic disciplines and a wide variety of theoretical and methodological perspectives. The series has a commitment to substantive problems and issues and favors research and analysis which seek to blend actual observations of human actions in daily life with broader theoretical, comparative, and historical perspectives. SOCIOLOGICAL OBSERVATIONS aims to use all of our available intellectual resources to better understand all facets of human experience and the nature of our society."

—John M. Johnson

Volumes in this series:

1. THE NUDE BEACH, by Jack D. Douglas and Paul K. Rasmussen, with Carol Ann Flanagan
2. SEEKING SPIRITUAL MEANING, by Joseph Damrell
3. THE SILENT COMMUNITY, by Edward William Delph
4. CROWDS AND RIOTS, by Sam Wright
5. THE MAD GENIUS CONTROVERSY, by George Becker
6. AMATEURS, by Robert A. Stebbins
7. CARETAKERS, by David R. Buckholdt and Jaber F. Gubrium
8. HARD HATS, by Jeffrey W. Reimer
9. LOVE AND COMMITMENT, by Gary Schwartz and Don Merten with Fran Behan and Allyne Rosenthal
10. OUTSIDERS IN A HEARING WORLD, by Paul C. Higgins
11. MOMENTUM, by Peter Adler
12. WORLDS OF FRIENDSHIP, by Robert R. Bell
13. CHRONIC PAIN, by Joseph A. Kotarba

CHRONIC PAIN

ITS SOCIAL DIMENSIONS

JOSEPH A. KOTARBA

foreword by
MARGO WYCKOFF

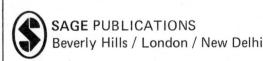
SAGE PUBLICATIONS
Beverly Hills / London / New Delhi

For information address:

SAGE Publications, Inc.
275 South Beverly Drive
Beverly Hills, California 90212

SAGE Publications India Pvt. Ltd.
C-236 Defence Colony
New Delhi 110 024, India

SAGE Publications Ltd
28 Banner Street
London EC1Y 8QE, England

Printed in the United States of America

Library of Congress Cataloging in Publication Data

Kotarba, Joseph A.
    Chronic pain.

    (Sociological observations ; 13)
    Bibliography: p.
    1. Pain—Social aspects. 2. Chronic diseases—
Social aspects. I. Title. II. Series. [DNLM:
1. Pain, Intractable. WL 704 K87c]
RB127.K67 1982   362.1'960472   82-16851
ISBN 0-8039-1880-1
ISBN 0-8039-1881-X (pbk.)

FIRST PRINTING

TO POLLY
my sweetheart

Contents

Acknowledgments 9

Foreword by Margo Wyckoff 11

1. Introduction 13
   Sociological Viewpoints 21

2. Medical and Paramedical Perspectives 27
   Medical Perspectives 28
   Paramedical Perspectives 36
     Nursing 37
     Clinical Psychology 42
     Medical Social Work 47
   Summary: Toward a Sociology of the Chronic
     Pain Experience 50

3. Becoming a Pain-Afflicted Person 55
   Stage I: The Onset of Pain 58
   Stage II: The Emergence of Doubt 64
   Stage III: The Chronic Pain Experience 71
   Conning the Physican 75
   Variations in the Chronic Pain Career 78
   The Family's Impact on the Search for a Cure 84

4. Complementary Health Care Modalities 91
   A Phenomenology of the Chiropractic Encounter 98
   Applied Mysticism 106
     Meditation 111
     Biofeedback and Autogenic Training 115
     Acupuncture 117
   The Chronic Pain Center 117
   Why Complementary Health Care Modalities? 129

5. "Play With Pain, Talk Injury": The Professional
   Athlete   133
   Talking About Pain   137
   The Athletic Subculture   151
   The Role of the Athletic Trainer   156
   Secrecy at Home   160
   Professional Sports Careers and Chronic Pain   162

6. "Play With Pain, Talk Injury": The Blue-Collar
   Manual Laborer   165
   Comparisons and Contrasts   167
   The Tavern Subculture   169
   Pain Control in the Tavern Setting   175
   Secrecy at Home: Talking "Faked" Injury   179
   Occupational Medicine and Chronic Pain   182

7. Physicians, Patients, and Pain: An Overview   185
   The Functionalist Model: Parsons's Sick Role   187
   The Marxist Model: Medicine as Business   191
   The Interactionist Model: The Social Construction
      of Illness   194
   The Decision-Making Model: The Rational Patient   197
   An Existential Model of the Chronic Pain Experience   199
   A Prospective Look at the Chronic Pain Phenomenon   204

References   209

About the Author   224

Acknowledgments

The idea for this study originated in 1974 during conversations with Dr. Peter Ortiz, a kind and thoughtful specialist in physical medicine and acupuncture. Dr. Ortiz not only facilitated my research on the emerging role of acupuncturists in the American health care system, but also encouraged me to explore the lives and experiences of the desperate people who flocked to his office daily with a mysterious affliction known as chronic pain. Since then, many others have assisted me along the way, and I would like to acknowledge their generosity.

My mentors at the University of California at San Diego—particularly Fred Davis, Joseph R. Gusfield, Bennett M. Berger, J. Anthony Deutsch, and Michael E. Parrish—were instrumental in the construction of the early drafts of this book. My colleagues have offered me the invaluable gifts of friendship and intellectual stimulation, especially David Altheide, Andy Fontana, Paul Rasmussen, James E. Hughes, June Lowenberg, Robert Snow, Peter Adler, Patti Adler, Margo McCaffery, John Seidel, Margo Wyckoff, Carol Warren, and Kathleen Ferraro. I will always cherish my afternoon discussions in sunny La Jolla with John Hund and Armando Arias, who helped me refine my sociological vision. Special thanks go to Jack Douglas and John Johnson for letting me share in their love for the social world.

I am most grateful to Mike Ryan (Public Information Officer, Houston Astros Baseball Club), Paul Lowenberg,

Richard Stieg, and Ed Wade for their assistance during the collection of data for the study. Material support for this work was provided in part by the National Research Service Award (NIH AA07129-01), the University of California Dissertation Research Award, the Kosciuszko Foundation Fellowship, and grants from the Center for Public Policy at the University of Houston. The faculty of sociology at the University of Houston generated much of the energy I needed to complete this work through their appreciation for the value of everyday-life sociology.

Above all, the very existence of this study is due to the many pain-afflicted people who believed in it. In return for their trust, honesty, and enthusiasm, I hope that this book will provide others with a better understanding of what it's like to live with chronic pain.

—J. K.

Foreword

Chronic pain is one of mankind's oldest afflictions, yet one of its least understood. Recent advances in research on basic pain mechanisms, innovative medical and pharmacological treatments, and the application of psychological and behavioral strategies have given hope to many sufferers. But countless more are untreated, maltreated, or overtreated. Above all, those of us who work directly with chronic pain patients have become increasingly aware of the widespread implications of their suffering—not only in the complex ways it affects virtually every aspect of their lives, but also in the impacts it has on all levels of the health care system. The message is clear: Effective mastery of the chronic pain phenomenon will require intense interdisciplinary efforts.

In this regard Professor Kotarba's book is a welcome addition to the literature. By taking a uniquely objective sociological stance, he can analyze critical elements of the chronic pain phenomenon that we tend to take for granted or ignore due to the overwhelmingly clinical orientation of pain work today. Professor Kotarba takes us through the emergent chronic pain career, as seen from the patient's perspective. We learn that the patient's primary goal in seeking healers is to find viable *meaning* in otherwise senseless suffering, meaning that will be sought from alternative sources if medicine proves inadequate to provide it. But we also get a glimpse of the more fundamental, existential dimensions of the chronic pain experience, how it affects one's daily activities and how it evokes feelings of irrationality, secrecy, fear, hope, and hopelessness.

As an administrator of a pain control center and a practicing psychologist, I find Professor Kotarba's discussion of professionalization among pain care workers intriguing. Effective pain care is not only the goal of our work; it is also a vehicle by which we can advance our disciplines and our personal careers. Thus Professor Kotarba reminds us of the responsibility inherent in the power we hold as sources of meaning for desperate patients.

In all, this book is must reading for anyone who is professionally or personally involved with the chronic pain phenomenon or with contemporary issues in health and illness. Social scientists especially will find this book fascinating, not only for its use of some very creative field research methods, but also for the new life it adds to our theoretical understanding of the physician/patient relationship. Rigorous studies like this, permeated by intellectual acuity and a deep concern for the plight of one's subjects, are requisites for the eventual solution to the puzzle of human suffering.

—Margo Wyckoff
Seattle, Washington

1

INTRODUCTION

This is a study of the social meanings of chronic pain. Chronic pain is an ongoing experience of embodied discomfort that fails either to heal naturally or to respond to normal forms of medical intervention. Most incidences of chronic pain are associated with specific physiological pathologies such as structural disorders in the spine (for example, a "slipped disc"), arthritis, postoperative complications, migraine headaches, neuralgia, and amputations ("phantom limb pain"). There are also conspicuous cases of what physicians refer to as "psychogenic pain," which have no discernible physiological cause. In itself chronic pain is rarely life threatening, although it can result in great suffering for the estimated 30 to 40 million Americans who must live with it (Shealy, 1974a). During the past two decades, alologists (specialists in the study and treatment of pain) have come to redefine chronic pain as a disease in its own right, contradicting previous notions of it as a symptom of disease. Indeed many pain experts (for example, Bonica, 1974) discuss the chronic pain phenomenon in epidemic terms in light of the apparently large population of pain-afflicted persons and the $40 to $50 billion estimated yearly cost of health care, drugs, disability compensation, and lost wages.

Much of the impetus for defining chronic pain as a medical problem in its own right came from the dramatic emergence of acupuncture in the United States during the early 1970s (see Kotarba, 1975). The mass media popularized this ancient Eastern form of healing largely in conjunction with President Nixon's widely acclaimed visit to China in 1972. Upon learning that acupuncture promised effective treatment for otherwise intractable pain, many chronic pain sufferers flocked to both qualified and unqualified practitioners in hope of finding a "cure" denied them by American medicine.

This dramatic and public emergence of long-term sufferers gave credence to the claim that *chronic pain is among medicine's greatest failures* (Melzack, 1973). After exhausting his or her repertoire of medical knowledge and skills, the typical frustrated physician could only direct the pain-afflicted person to "learn to live with the pain," simultaneously trying to temper the discomfort with analgesic drugs.

Heavy reliance on analgesic drugs is likely, however, simply to reshape the chronic pain problem in two pernicious ways. First, the pain-afflicted person can inadvertently develop a physically and emotionally debilitating dependency on these drugs. Second, analgesic drugs tend to lose their effectiveness over time and actually increase the sensation of discomfort.

Thus many perceived acupuncture not only as a source of pain relief, but also as a potentially harmless substitute for noxious drug dependency (Kotarba, 1975: 173). The popularization of acupuncture hinted of the complexity, as well as the magnitude, of the chronic pain phenomenon.

The essence of the everyday reality of the chronic pain experience and the quality of that experience that distinguishes it from most other health problems is the existential nature of the affliction. Chronic pain is inherently private and remains unnoticed by others unless actively disclosed by the sufferer. We cannot easily perceive another's pain as we could observe a broken limb, paralysis, or an infectious disease. People afflicted with chronic pain in the absence of other afflictions or disabilities appear quite normal, because chronic pain has no visible pathology. Chronic pain also knows no age barriers. We might expect certain elderly people to be in pain simply because of our commonsense understanding of the aging process, but we do not ordinarily expect a young and otherwise healthy-looking person to be experiencing protracted pain with little hope for a cure. With the exception of those relatively few people who become functionally disabled due to the severity of their pain, most pain-afflicted people continue to present what we perceive as "normal" physiological identities.

In order to understand the private nature of chronic pain, it is useful to compare it with acute pain, the more common form of physical discomfort. Acute pain acts as a warning that something, usually interpreted as tissue damage, is wrong with the body. An unexpected, sharp sensation of pain elicits a reflex response, which may either be verbal ("ouch") or gesticulatory (a grimace or limp). If the pain is caused by an external stimulus, such as a blow or connection with a sharp object, the body reflexively retacts away from the harmful agent. These pain behaviors are indications to others that one is hurting. Chronic pain, on the other hand, ordinarily does not elicit reflex responses. Defensive reflexes diminish over time, because they do not help. The pain will persist no matter what the person may do to try to ease it. Through habituation, chronic pain becomes a benign and expected physical experience no longer requiring an outward display. Whereas acute pain is more or less an embodied crisis in the forefront of one's attention and display of self, chronic pain is largely a routine background feature of everyday experience (see Sternbach, 1974: 5-7).

Why do we treat such an apparently individualistic and biological experience as a *sociological* phenomenon? The answer lies in the pain-afflicted person's response to the physician's common prescription, "Learn to live with the pain." Living with chronic pain means coping, and *coping is an inherently social enterprise* in two distinct ways. First and foremost, pain-afflicted people almost never resign themselves to blind and passive acceptance of their suffering. They reach out to others for viable meanings for the pain. Their most pressing need is for effective medical diagnosis they hope will lead to a cure or at least reasonable control of the pain. Their search for healing may result in "doctor hopping" in the attempt to locate the "right" physician or the "right" cure. At the point when they perceive normal medicine as inadequate, now increasingly desperate pain-afflicted persons are likely to experiment with a plethora of nonmedical health care nostrums that still seem to offer hope. But ultimately, when health care workers of any sort cannot give meaning to this seemingly endless suffering, the pain-afflicted person may search for a transcendental context for the pain. Religion is a common source of this understanding, proposing chronic pain as either a punishment or a reward for mere human existence, or perhaps as a rite of passage into some higher form of being.

Second, chronic pain is a fairly *constant* experience of discomfort. This constancy means that it accompanies its sufferer in all social situations. The invisibility of chronic pain provides the pain-afflicted person with a certain amount of discretion in deciding whether or not to allow the pain to become a relevant topic in any interaction. Inherent privacy thus becomes situational secrecy. For example, pain-afflicted people will reveal the pain to health care workers in order to receive treatment, and to friends and family members in order to receive sympathy, support, and understanding. But these same people will conceal the pain if they judge its revelation to be potentially damaging to their better interests, as is often the case in occupations—such as professional sports and blue-collar labor—where job security rests on high levels of physical competence. On a more intimate level, the pain-afflicted may decide to conceal the fact that vigorous sexual activity increases the sensation of pain if they see this disclosure as potentially damaging to their sexual identities.

This book explores the ways individuals cope with chronic pain across various types of relevant social situations. I hope the data and analysis presented here will serve both *informational* and *theoretical* purposes. Although there is an extensive (and growing) body of scientific/medical literature on the mechanisms of pain per se, very little is commonly known about the everyday experience of chronic pain. What information we have is mostly concerned with and based on the actualization and management of pain within medical settings or the psychological traits of pain-afflicted people as measured by clinically administered and interpreted personality inventories. This book elaborates on this knowledge by describing the more routine features of the chronic pain experience within the natural situations of everyday life, especially at work and in the family. In addition, by taking a sociological (as opposed to a clinical) view toward chronic pain, we can appreciate the multidimensional nature of the pain-afflicted person's search for help.

Chapter 2 will review the medical and paramedical perspectives on chronic pain. It discusses the importance of chronic pain to various health care occupations within the context of the process of professionalization. Organized medicine, the dominant form of health care in our society, has traditionally responded to both acute and chronic pain with surgery and drugs. The glaring failure of these approaches in alleviating chronic pain has given many professionally aspiring members of the paramedical occupations—specifically nursing, clinical psychology, and medical social work—the opportunity to claim expertise in this area in their efforts to achieve higher status in the health care system.

Chapter 3 describes the psychosocial process of becoming a pain-afflicted person, seen through the perspective of the patient. The two contrasting themes in the emergence of a chronic pain career are the *clinical* and the *experiential.* Clinically, the medical evaluation of a pain condition progresses in a straight line from acute to chronic. Experientially, the pain-afflicted person always attempts to maintain a sense of control over the pain, which is only situationally effective, yet refuses to accept the inevitability of endless suffering denoted by the term "chronic." Put differently, the feeling of hope that interweaves through the chronic pain experience is a prime reason for the continuous active search for a cure.

I have decided to portray the process of becoming a pain-afflicted person in one unitary career model, as opposed to constructing several models that might indicate variations in the process resulting from the social, economic, and cultural characteristics of the subjects. My reasons for this are based upon the nature of the phenomenon. During the course of this research, I became increasingly aware of the striking *similarities* among chronic pain experiences. In analyzing case after case, I learned of the same initial definition of acuteness, the same disillusionment with medicine as the problem persisted unabated, the same decision to seek help outside normal medicine, and so on. Thus it seemed wise, first, to pursue a comprehensive understanding of the essence of the chronic pain experience and then to deal with certain key variations as separate topics.

Chapter 4 discusses the use of complementary health care modalities (CHCM), such as chiropractic, naturopathy, acupuncture, and religion. CHCM become viable alternatives to medicine at that point in the career when the sufferer determines that medicine has been ineffective in managing the pain. I argue that alternative forms of health care are complementary to medicine because the vast majority of their patients, seeking help for pain problems, utilize them in search of specific therapeutic goals while maintaining belief in the *overall* efficacy of medicine. Several new forms of CHCM, such as hypnosis, meditation, and autogenic training, fall under the rubric of *applied mysticism,* which is the promotion of transcendental or metaphysical belief systems for pain control through "higher" states of consciousness. The emergence of the chronic pain center demonstrates the institutionalization of CHCM in settings conducive to the medical model of pain care. Crucial to an understanding of CHCM is the fact that pain-afflicted people of *all* social backgrounds use CHCM, although variations in social status largely determine which CHCM may be consulted.

Chapter 5 describes the occupational relevance of chronic pain to the careers of professional athletes, using the more general context of the athletic injury. The commonly used expression "play with pain, talk injury" (PWP, TI) neatly summarizes the dilemma faced by many athletes in deciding whether or not to disclose nonvisible pain to potentially critical audiences (management, the press, and the fans). An athlete ordinarily will obtain assistance in making this decision and in developing strategies for coping with pain through involvement with the athletic subculture. In addition I will explore ways in which the team trainer acts as mediator between the athlete and the audiences to his or her work in the establishment of meaning for athletic injury and pain.

Chapter 6 applies the expression "PWP, TI" in its generic sense to blue-collar labor—another occupational category for which physical competence is a requisite for job success. Although the motivation among manual laborers to conceal pain-related problems is considerably weaker than that of professional athletes, certain contingencies like potential loss of self-esteem or job advancement may lead these workers to conceal pain from their own critical audiences (spouses or foremen). The tavern subculture provides assistance to many of these workers through the dissemination of health care information and the availability of alcoholic beverages as folk analgesics.

Chapter 7 summarizes the study and provides an analysis of the impact of the findings on the sociological understanding of the physician/patient relationship. The four major models in the literature provide one-sided perspectives by emphasizing either the paternalistic, economic, priestly, or rationalist aspects of this relationship. In the case of the chronic pain experience, however, the *essence* of this relationship lies not in any single, categorical dimension, but is found in the way each dimension waxes and wanes in importance over the course of a lengthy and uncertain condition. Patterns of change occurring in the overall conduct of the relationship strongly reflect transformations in the patient's definition of the strengths and weaknesses of specific encounters with healers. In turn the very possibility of patient autonomy in redefining the relationship is linked with transformations in self-concept that occur during the course of the search for meaning.

A comment on the *tone* of this study is in order at this juncture. This book depicts numerous criticisms of medicine and the medical management of chronic pain, emanating from other health care workers and especially from the pain-afflicted people themselves. These negative viewpoints are not a rationale for some sort of "political" attack against the institution of medicine, but are an attempt to remain true to the emotionally charged phenomenon of chronic pain. Many people find it quite difficult to reconcile the dissonance between organized medicine's economic, political, and cultural preeminence in our society and its inability to effectively deal with pain. Many pain-afflicted people are intensely angry because their high expectations for the power of medicine were cruelly shattered. Whether or not these criticisms are in some objective way true is beyond the scope of this book and the province of sociology. The sociological task is to look beyond blaming the problem of chronic pain on any one thing and to arrive at an understanding of the *nature* of human suffering and the dynamics of socially organized coping mechanisms.

SOCIOLOGICAL VIEWPOINTS

Theoretically, this study confronts several key conceptual issues in the sociology of health and illness. The chronic pain phenomenon is relevant to the *process of professionalization* occurring within the health care world today. Members of several paramedical occupations, such as nursing and clinical psychology, have claimed expertise in the treatment of chronic pain as a vehicle for ascendancy into the ranks of the true professional, a status traditionally occupied solely by the physician in the realm of health care. On another level the chronic pain experience enlightens our understanding of the *nature of the physician/patient relationship.* This study provides data on the highly emotional, often conflict-ridden, and occasionally irritational forms this relationship can assume. Existing sociological models of this relationship do not adequately account for the complexity of the physician/ patient interaction, a shortcoming I hope to alleviate in this study.

The major theoretical topic addressed in this study, though, is the *process of the individual's search for meaning during experiences of embodied distress.* I am indebted for insight into the nature of social meanings to three theoretical perspectives in sociological thought that together form the nucleus of "everyday-life sociology": symbolic interactionism, phenomenological sociology, and existential sociology.

Symbolic interactionism was the first sociological perspective to seriously consider social meanings as the essence of social life. According to Blumer's (1969) distinctive summary of this position, human beings act toward things on the basis of the meanings these things have for them. Meanings arise out of the social interaction one engages in with others. Above all, meanings are handled and modified through an ongoing process of interpretation and application. The "things" to which Blumer refers can be any objects that strike one's attention. In this study the thing being made sense of its intractable pain, and the "others" are the lay and professional sources of help.

Phenomenological sociology focuses upon the *cognitive* aspects of meaning construction—that is, the ways language and consciousness allow us to display a sense of social order to ourselves and to each other (see Psathas, 1973). Accordingly, conversation not only relays information about phenomena such as chronic pain, but also creates an intersubjective world in which social phenomena are made possible for its members. Throughout this study, I illustrate some of the mechanisms of "pain talk" by which this most private of experiences is put into words. The pain talk in the conversational milieu of the blue-collar tavern, which we will explore in Chapter 6, is a good example of this phenomenon.

The emerging field of *existential sociology* has been the most important theoretical influence on this study. The principal writers in this perspective (for example, Kotarba, 1979; Douglas and Johnson, 1977) argue that effective social science must begin with an understanding of how members actually *experience* social life in concrete, everyday-life situations. Within the context of one's total experience of the world, social meanings are meshed with feelings, creativity, and even episodes of meaninglessness or absurdity. This perspective lends itself well to the study of chronic pain behavior because of the immense difficulty pain-afflicted people have in "making sense of" their physical distress.

The social meanings generated during the course of coping with chronic pain serve two purposes. First, the pain-afflicted person incurs meaning for the pain itself from various others. The effectiveness of these lay and professional diagnoses— that is, the degree to which these meanings are adopted by the pain-afflicted person—is mediated and constrained by the ontological reality of the pain. *The precognitive, embodied reality of chronic pain is preeminent and cannot readily be defined away symbolically.* For this reason, the pain-afflicted person will commonly reject diagnoses that do not "fit" the experience of pain, imply that the pain is not "real" by indicating a psychological cause for the discomfort (for instance, psychosomia), or do not lead to effective treatment. In these situations the search for meaning continues.

Second, social meanings serve to define the pain-afflicted person's very being—or self. Since the sufferer faces uncertain resolution of the dilemma, the experience of coping with chronic pain has implications for the individual's occupational and interpersonal relationships and, therefore, self-esteem and social status. In order to preserve self-esteem, the sick person attempts to present his or her condition correctly to others in interaction, according to the norms of face-to-face interaction in effect in each particular social situation. Davis (1961) describes the process of *deviance disavowal* by which visibly handicapped persons like the blind and facially disfigured normalize their conditions by separating their "true selves" from the socially/morally discrediting handicap. Through movement from the establishment of fictional

acceptance of normalcy to the projection of a self that adequately performs normal social roles, the visibly handicapped person eliminates the handicap as a potentially
embarrassing or burdensome relevance to interaction.

Elaborating upon Davis's analysis, the present study
focuses upon the formal and informal rules that organize the
display of *competency* in coping with chronic pain. In situations in which pain-afflicted persons disclose their suffering
to others, they feel obliged to demonstrate that they are
reacting properly to their condition. Competent pain-afflicted
persons, for example, demonstrate emotional control over
the pain, even when in their own minds they feel that they are
not coping well, and talk about their doctors as being the
"best" available practitioners, even when they personally
feel little confidence in the effectiveness of their doctors.
Competency is also directed toward health care workers
through techniques ranging from requests for help, as opposed
to demands for a cure, to the display of faithful diligence to
prescribed exercises whether or not these exercises are in
fact undertaken. These displays of competence may be representative, in a generic sense, of the presentations of self
that occur in any illness.

I have chosen to examine the chronic pain phenomenon
through a multiperspectival approach to field research. As
Douglas (1976: 189-197) argues, it is important to understand the perspectives of all groups relevant to complex
social phenomena, and chronic pain is no exception. In this
study I contrast the perspectives of health care workers with
that of the patient in order to explain the almost inevitable
conflict that arises over the management of chronic pain.
Since the professional perspectives on chronic pain are well
documented in literature, I paid special attention to the
patient's perspective during my investigation, especially the
pain-afflicted person's knowledge and evaluation of health
care options. This is not to imply that the subject is totally or

even meaningfully aware of the normative constraints shaping his or her patterns of coping, or that the subject's evaluation of pain care—which is often quite negative—is definitive in any objective, let alone scientific, sense. The pain-afflicted person's definition of the situation, though, has real consequences for the course of his or her pain career. For example, the irrational fear of surgery leads many pain-afflicted people to resort to nonsurgical types of intervention like chiropractic, even when surgery is perceived medically as the only proper treatment.

I collected data for this study through a variety of field research techniques, most notably participant observation, formal interviews, and informal conversations.[1] The exploratory nature of the study and the amorphous nature of the chronic pain experience required my reliance upon the strategy of *discovering* representative subjects and settings. Due to the pervasiveness and secrecy of chronic pain in our society, which I learned through my earlier research on the social organization of acupuncture (Kotarba, 1977, 1975), I realized that it would be impossible to establish valid parameters a priori for the entire population of helpers and help seekers. I also could not expect the subjects present within any particular health care setting to represent the entire population of pain-afflicted persons because of the apparent existence of many sufferers who rarely if ever seek "formal" health care for their pain. I therefore decided to defocus my search for various chronic pain experiences and to be open to discoveries in all walks of life and in all segments of the community. By submerging myself into the everyday-life social world and attempting to be a competent member in tune with the nuances of that world, I encountered numerous people who either experience chronic pain themselves or know of others who do.

I used three general types of resources for collecting data: the community, the university, and strictly personal contacts. Community resources included (among others) local hospitals, chronic pain centers, alternative health care practitioners, and YMCA exercise classes. The local media, which regularly carry feature stories on this now popular topic, provided valuable information on available pain-care services. As a member of the academic community, I was surrounded by a wealth of pain-related resources. I encountered a number of pain-afflicted people at Siddah Yoga and chronic pain seminars sponsored by the university's extension service. The university's public information officer became my primary contact with professional athletes, for whom chronic pain is a distinct occupational concern. My involvement with a drinking/driving research project put me in direct contact with the local tavern subculture and its role in helping blue-collar laborers cope with job-related injuries and pain. Finally, friends and acquaintances have been especially useful in locating pain-afflicted people who rarely consult healers but rely heavily on self-care, a common situation among the elderly.

NOTE

1. Kotarba (1980b) provides a detailed account of the methods and natural history of this study. Of particular relevance is my discussion of contacts and their usefulness in helping me gain entree to difficult settings and in raising important empirical questions.

2

MEDICAL AND
PARAMEDICAL PERSPECTIVES

There is little doubt that organized medicine is the dominant form of health care in the United States. As such it not only maintains nearly total control over its own work, but it also largely defines the work domains of its paramedical assistants (Friedson, 1970). The theoretical approaches to and the clinical management of chronic pain reflect this power relationship. In this chapter I will first discuss the medical perspective on chronic pain and demonstrate how medicine's scientific/Cartesian paradigm, which has served it so well in controlling many other types of disease, limits its effectiveness in managing chronic pain. Then I will discuss the ways in which some ambitious paramedics use their particular claims to expertise in treating chronic pain as vehicles for potential admission to the ranks of the true health care professional, a position traditionally held only by the physician in our society.

MEDICAL PERSPECTIVES

Medical views of pain in general, and of chronic pain in particular, have remained faithful to historical developments in the Western theory of illness and disease.[1] As Ritzer (1975), Kuhn (1970), and others have persuasively argued, all sciences work within the constraints of their respective models, or paradigms. A paradigm is a taken-for-granted framework specifying the appropriate problems for investigation, the appropriate methods of inquiry, and the criteria for drawing inferences from facts to more general, abstract, or theoretical statements. In other words a paradigm reflects the "textbook" state of a science governing everyday research and problem solving.

The history of modern medicine depicts the development of a scientific paradigm for healing based on systematic, detached observation of the body and its functions (DuBos, 1969). Just as Copernicus had displaced man and his world from the center of the universe, modern practitioners of medicine displace the analysis of *suffering* and all its metaphysical and religious connotations with an analysis of the body as a *machine* for which observable *causes* for disease could be discerned. In this light pain is no longer viewed as a curse of God, as it was often written of in the Old Testament, nor as a natural result of original sin, as the New Testament stated.[2] Pain has increasingly come to be seen as an indicator of bodily malfunctioning, a signal of physical pathology to be located and explained through the scientific method.

Descartes presented the first "scientific" theory of pain in 1644.[3] The mechanical metaphor that served Descartes so well in describing the nature of the cosmos became a means of treating the body as an *object*. In Illich's (1976: 150) words:

[Descartes] constructed an image of the body in terms of geometry, mechanics, or watchmaking, a machine that could be repaired by an engineer. The body became an apparatus owned and managed by the soul, but from an almost infinite distance. The living body experience which the French refer to as "la Chair" and the Germans as "der Leib" was reduced to a mechanism that the soul could inspect.

Descartes viewed pain as a signal by which the body reacted to imminent danger to its mechanical integrity. Pain followed a pathway that directly linked the skin with the brain. Like the bell-ringing mechanism in a church, in which a man pulls the rope at the bottom of the tower and the bell rings in the belfry, pain felt within an extremity served as a warning signal to the soul that danger was imminent. The Creator, in His ultimate wisdom, made pain as a sort of negatively reinforcing learning device to protect the body from harm, as occurs when you pulled your hand away from an open flame because you perceived that the flame's heat was a warning (see Melzack, 1973: 126-127).

Descartes's simplistic notion of pain as a distinct activity of the sensory system was more or less unquestioned by Western medicine for the next 250 years. During that time, physicians still relied on the effectiveness of opium, henbane, and a few other natural drugs for the relief of pain in much the same way as had the Egyptians, Chinese, and Greeks hundreds of years earlier. It was not until the Listerian era, the nineteenth century, that physicians could attempt surgically to sever Descartes's hypothetical pathways of pain without fear of infection (Bonica, 1953: 20-22). The emergence of the experimental science of physiology in the mid-nineteenth century sensitized researchers to a new problem: How do we account for variations in sensations (such as smell as compared to touch) as well as in levels of pain? Von Frey developed Descartes's basic notions in modern physiological terms with his pronouncement of the *specificity theory of pain* in 1894 (Melzack, 1973: 129; Melzack and Wall, 1965). Von Frey argued that there are specific pain receptors (free nerve endings), which, when stimulated, result in the sensation of pain. Painful stimuli are transferred along a unique set of peripheral nerves to the brain, where they are automatically interpreted as pain. The pain receptors and peripheral nerves are totally different from the structures in body tissue related to other sensations such as touch, warmth, and cold.[4]

In the same year Von Frey formulated his theory, Goldschneider proposed an alternative *pattern theory of pain* (Melzack, 1973: 139-147; Fordyce, 1976: 14-15). In light of clinical evidence showing that there was no one-to-one relationship between pain perception and the intensity of the stimulus, Goldschneider argued that the sensation of pain resulted from special patterns of stimuli intensity and interpretation in the brain, and no specific nerve endings were needed to transmit impulses. Pain resulted when the total output of skin sensory cells exceeded a critical level, caused either by excessive stimulation of sense receptors or pathological conditions that enhanced the impulses produced by normally nonnoxious stimuli.

Goldschneider's theory was directed toward explaining two types of clinically induced pain. First, there was often a delay between the onset of stimuli and the actual sensation of pain, as when a pinprick is not felt until many seconds later. Second, patients suffering from certain pathological conditions like *tabes dorsalis* often felt tremendous pain after the application of gentle pressure or mild heat. Later refinements of pattern theory contended that transmitted impulse patterns were also affected by other central nervous system imputs on a psychological level, such as variable emotional states, the individual's prior experience with pain, situational mental alertness, and the like (Fordyce, 1976: 14).

The specificity theory of pain, along with its refinements, has dominated medical thought and practice ever since. It is still being taught in most medical schools (in some cases as the *only* theory of pain) and forms the basis for the discussion of pain in most medical textbooks (Melzack, 1973: 126;

Fordyce, 1976: 14). It has proved to be a powerful theory, giving rise to important research and some effective forms of pain treatment, and there are three underlying, *paradigmatic* reasons for its general acceptance by physicians. First, specificity theory fits the "one disease/one cause" perspective of traditional Western medicine. The effectiveness of the germ theory of disease, which led to the discovery of specific microorganisms responsible for various diseases, has organized medical thinking toward simple explanations of disease and physiological functions. Pattern theory, on the other hand, has often been criticized for not being sufficiently anatomically exact (Casey, 1973).

Second, specificity theory is conducive to the traditional emphasis on surgical intervention in disease. Pattern theory proposes only vague patterns of pain mechanisms that the surgeon cannot easily locate (Melzack, 1973: 150).

Third, the components of specificity theory are strictly physiological, whereas pattern theory suggests the importance of psychological factors in the pain experience. This particular aspect of pattern theory runs contrary to medicine's traditional goal of locating and treating physiological causes for physiological problems.

Both chemical and surgical techniques can be based on specificity theory. Analgesics like codeine, Demerol, and morphine can chemically depress the central nervous system at the thalamus and the cerebral cortex and thus interrupt and alter the perception of pain. Other chemical agents such as saline solutions can work as nerve blocks to interrupt the transmission of pain in the dorsal and peripheral nerve areas, much like the effect of novocaine injection on tooth pain. Surgical techniques can sever the nerve path itself. While the general use of this kind of surgically induced lesions is presently in disfavor due to the high risk of paralysis and, in the case of lobotomies, dehumanization, surgery is still a very common procedure for the relief of low-back pain. Between 50,000 and 75,000 Americans undergo spinal disc surgery every year (Freese, 1974: 30; see also Bonica, 1953).

While medicine has been most effective in the management of *acute* pain, as exemplified by the accomplishments of modern anesthesiology, it has been notoriously ineffective with *chronic* pain (Bonica, 1953; Melzack, 1973; Mines, 1974; Sternbach, 1974; Leroy, 1977). The long-term use of narcotic analgesic drugs often leads to habituation and drug abuse (Fordyce, 1976: 157). Laminectomy, the most widespread type of surgery for disc pathologies, is totally effective less than 50 percent of the time (Shealy, 1974a: 133). The most glaring example of the weakness of medical theory and practice in dealing with pain is in treatment of the phantom limb phenomenon (Melzack, 1973: 50-60). Most amputees report feeling a phantom limb soon after the amputation of an arm or a leg (Simmel, 1956). In most cases pain associated with the phantom limb disappears in time, but in approximately 5 to 10 percent the pain is severe and may grow worse (Feinstein et al., 1954), even in patients with perfectly healed stumps. This problem is relatively rare among war amputees, who tend to lose a limb suddenly. It is more common among civilian amputees with histories of pain in the previously diseased limb. If the specificity theory of pain were valid, then the loss of the limb and its accompanying nerve supply would result in the loss of all sensation in the area. Additional surgery to sever nerve channels from the stump to the sensory cortex (the area of the brain to which nerve impulses are projected) routinely fail to alleviate the pain.[5]

A scientific paradigm remains secure until the persistence of unexplained anomalies leads to crisis (Kuhn, 1970: 66-76). Novel theories then emerge to solve the puzzles not accounted for by *normal* science. Recently medicine has not only become increasingly aware of its own ineffectiveness in treating chronic pain, but has witnessed the spread of seemingly effective nonmedical treatments like acupuncture and hypnosis. A major breakthrough in the solution of this dilemma came in 1965 when Melzack and Wall, two neurophysiological researchers, published their *gate control theory of pain*. They tried to incorporate the useful elements of both specificity and pattern theory into a single model that would explain all aspects of pain and its treatment.

In their discussion of existing theories, Melzack and Wall "considered it important to recognize the obvious physiologic specialization of the nervous system without accepting the narrow specificity of such terms as 'pain receptors' and 'pain pathway,' which imply a rigid one-to-one relationship between input and the eventual psychologic experience" (Melzack, 1977: 80). Specificity theory is not only inadequate to explain why cutting a nerve does not always abolish pain below the cut, but also ignores *emotional* factors affecting the pain experience. For example, Hill et al. (1952) found that subjects experiencing experimentally induced anxiety feel electric shock or burning heat to be more painful. Pattern theory's notion of pain as a simple and direct relationship between the severity of the external noxious stimulus and the level of pain response ignores the role played by cognitive and psychological processes. Melzack and Wall cited Beecher's (1959) classic study of American soldiers who sustained injuries at Anzio in World War II. A significant number of soldiers sustaining obvious tissue damage from combat wounds nevertheless reported little or no pain because of the perceived benefits of their injuries. their wounds were seen as a way out of their continued life-threatening presence at the front.

Briefly, the gate control theory postulates the existence of physiological gates that can swing shut to selectively block out pain. These hypothetical gates would be located in the gray matter of the spinal cord, the *substantia gelantinosa,* where the peripheral nerve fibers enter and are jointed with the central transmission fibers to the brain. If a stimulus is applied to the skin, both the large nerve fibers, supposed to carry the sensation of touch, and the small nerve fibers, supposed to carry the sensation of pain, respond. When the brain is bombarded by impulses from the small nerve fibers, the person feels pain. Melzack and Wall argue, however, that the pain impulses can be reduced or eliminated by means of several inhibitory mechanisms. First, the large nerve fibers on the surface of the skin can be stimulated by vibration, scratching, or rubbing to cause the brain to "close the gates." This sort of thing commonly occurs when you bang your elbow against a piece of furniture. Your immediate reaction is to rub the injured spot, which loads the large fibers, causing the brain to signal to close the gate, and the messages of pain from the small nerve fibers are terminated. The application of warmth to a minor cut acts the same way. Second, the brain stem—the "pain center" of the entire body, according to Melzack and Wall's theory—can be stimulated to close various gates by the interaction of cognitive, emotional, experiential, or suggestive factors.

The gate control theory has succeeded in calling great attention to chronic pain "as a medical syndrome in its own right, rather than merely a symptom of other pathological processes" (Melzack, 1977: 89). Possibly the most important aspect of the theory and its supporting research is the emphasis it places on the powerful descending control of the higher nervous system over the gate. In terms of chronic pain, *depression,* for example, has been found to situationally reinforce and even *cause* pain in the absence of external noxious stimuli (Melzack and Chapman, 1973). The gate control theory also offers plausible explanations for the effectiveness of certain nontraditional pain therapies. The implanting of acupuncture needles may interrupt the transmission of pain impulses by stimulating large nerve fibers on the skin surface to close the gate (Melzack, 1973: 185-190).[6] The *voluntary* stimulation of the brain to close the gate may explain the effectiveness of biofeedback, self-hypnosis, meditation, and other forms of autosuggestion

(Melzack and Chapman, 1973; Hilgard, 1978). Finally, there is a growing body of neurophysiological research exploring the relationship between the gating mechanism and the body's self-made pain killers, the *endorphins*. Cheng and Pomeranz (1979) were able to reduce chronic pain experimentally by implanting electrodes in the brain stem and electrically stimulating the gray matter to release endorphins. They argue that the endorphins then attach to certain opiate receptors such as acupuncture points, trigger points, and pain gates to block incoming pain signals (see also Cannon et al., 1978; Costa and Trabucchi, 1978).

In spite of these dramatic developments in the theory and practice of pain relief, medicine has been slow in adopting them into regular health work. Any normal science is basically *conservative* and tries to solve all puzzles or anomalies within its existing theoretical and methodological frameworks (Kuhn, 1970: 111-134). Revolutions in science occur only when a competing paradigm is sufficiently powerful to replace the basic assumptions of the science and to cause scientists to radically alter their perceptions of the world. Medicine, for the most part, has remained both theoretically and clinically skeptical to the new approaches to pain evolving from the gate control theory (Brimble, 1979; Crue in Mines, 1974: 15-19). Most physicians still rely on traditional modes of pain treatment which, though unsatisfactory in treating chronic pain, remain true to the overall medical perspective. Since the medical paradigm has led to spectacular advances in so many areas of health care, especially in the control of infectious disease,[7] its proponents maintain that it will soon solve the "puzzle of pain" (Melzack, 1973) without lending credence to the unorthodox approaches that question medicine's core assumption of mind/body dualism (see Sovak, 1979).

To the contrary, however, many *behavior-oriented* paraprofessional health workers use the newly discovered cognitive, emotional, and situational aspects of pain to provide the rationale for treating chronic pain in ways that often differ greatly from medical prescription.

PARAMEDICAL PERSPECTIVES

If we were to imagine the role of the physician at the center of the health care system in America, then the paramedics would occupy the immediate periphery. Due to historic and technological advancements, a hierarchy of labor has developed around the work of the physician. The paramedical occupations have traditionally exhibited relatively little autonomy, prestige, or authority compared with medicine, since their work is ultimately controlled by physicians (Freidson, 1970: 47-52; see also Bliss and Cohen, 1977). Recently, however, some paramedics have pushed for professional status, due mostly to rising expectations of reward for their services and the perceived maldistribution, increased specialization, and rising cost of physician services (Freidson, 1970: 53-54; Coe, 1978: 244-256). In order to achieve higher recognition for their workers, the paramedical occupations must develop parameters for *domains of expertise,* separate from those of the physician, yet responsive to the needs of the health care market. Three paramedical specialties—nursing, clinical psychology, and medical social work—have incorporated chronic pain management into their domains.

Paraprofessional claims to expertise in the management of chronic pain reflect a shift in clinical concern from "pain" to the "pain patient" (Sternbach, 1974: 1-4). By definition, chronic pain is *intractable*—that is, it cannot be cured by normal medical intervention. In many cases medicine can only hope to *control* the pain as much as possible while helping the patients to learn to live with their pain and minimize its disruption of everyday activities and responsibilities. Physicians, as a group, are badly prepared to deal with these behavioral aspects of the chronic pain experience because of the largely self-imposed limitations of their profession. The "disease-oriented" or "acute care" model is dominant in American medicine (Fagerhaugh and Strauss, 1977: v), so that the typical physician has neither the time, the training, nor the patience to provide the long-term, interactive care required by chronic illness (Coe, 1978: 83). Instead, the labor-intensive care for chronic illness has been delegated to (or "dumped on," according to some health care workers) the paramedical occupations. In turn, some members of the paramedical occupations have used their expertise in the care of chronic illness to help fill the void created by growing disillusionment with medical approaches to chronic pain.

I will discuss nursing, clinical psychology, and medical social work perspectives on chronic pain in light of (1) their organizational and philosophical relationships with medicine; (2) their particular "humanistic" orientations to serving the ill; and (3) their particular use of the gate control theory as a theoretical foundation for professional advancement. Although other paramedical workers like pharmacists and physical therapists do come into contact with chronic pain patients, I limit my discussion to these three specialties because they have been especially interested in chronic pain and go beyond the mere execution of physicians' orders. They have begun the establishment of separate treatment methods.[8]

Nursing

Nursing is without question the most widespread and influential of the paramedical occupations.[9] There are approximately 820,000 persons employed as licensed registered nurses and another 500,000 employed as practical nurses in the United States (National Center for Health Statistics, 1980), representing the largest single group of health workers. Nurses rank second only to physicians in status and prestige among health workers (Cockerham, 1978: 147).

Nurses also work most closely with physicians in providing primary patient care and in assisting in administering drugs, surgery, and so on. Medical dominance in America has left nurses "in the role of a supporting cast" (Twaddle and Hessler, 1977: 188) whose primary duty is the fulfillment of doctors' orders. Occupational subservience is reinforced by the fact that over two-thirds of all nurses work in hospitals and related institutions controlled by physicians (Mauksch, 1972: 217). Thus nurses have not only had to carry out the decisions of physicians, but also adapt to the bureaucratic dictates of highly complex medical organizations.

Nursing's response to pain in general reflects this occupational dependency. For example, an orthopedic surgeon may diagnose a case of severe low-back pain as caused by a ruptured lumbar disc. If the surgeon decides that a laminectomy is required, the operating room nurse's duty is to assist in the performance of the operation. The ward nurse is obliged to administer postoperative analgesics according to the physician's prescription. If, on the other hand, the orthopedist decides in favor of a more conservative treatment, the ward nurse is required to organize and administer a regimen of, say, physical therapy and traction. In other words, the physician's perspective on pain and its application to particular patients largely shapes the nurse's active response to those patients (Strauss, 1966). While it is true that nurses can and often do influence the physician's decision making through what Stein (1967) refers to as the "doctor/nurse game," the fact that this negotiation must be subtle and kept on the level of the nurse's *recommendation* simply reinforces the ultimate authority of the physician.

The organizational settings of hospitals and clinics also affect nurses' management of pain, and especially of chronic pain. Medicine's "acute care" model permeates the formal and informal organization of health care facilities controlled by physicians. In any acute care hospital, a large percentage of patients must suffer the discomforts associated with surgery. In the course of routinizing their work, the staff typify patients according to certain "expected pain trajectories"

(Fagerhaugh and Strauss, 1977: 22) that arise from the staff's repeated experience with similar cases. The most commonly attributed pain trajectory is acute and directly related to the surgical process:

> On surgical wards . . . patients commonly arrive with some pain or no pain; after surgery they will be sedated through a few hours or days of considerable pain; and then, providing no complications arise, the pain will drop off at a rate appropriate to the type of surgery [Fagerhaugh and Strauss 1977: 22].

Chronic pain patients, on the other hand, present unpredictable and problematic pain trajectories. The staff, and especially the nurses who most come into contact with the patients, may become frustrated when a patient's pain does not diminish as expected. Nurse/patient interaction becomes strained and communication breaks down as the patient is labeled "uncooperative" or "difficult," while the nurse is labeled "uncaring" or "incompetent." In addition the nursing management of the chronic pain patient may be inherently flawed because the staff is unfamiliar with the patient's often lengthy history of pain, existing use of analgesic drugs, related emotional/psychological problems, and so on (Fagerhaugh and Strauss, 1977: 23-24).

Another essential aspect of nursing's approach to chronic pain is its view of its own ideology and goals. Nursing has traditionally been service oriented, professing the strong, humanitarian goal of relieving the suffering of the patient (Brown, 1975: 173-184). Within the everyday work setting, the nurse's management of pain involves not only the administering of doctor-ordered interventions, but also the comforting of patients by "imparting positive strength, hope, and cheer" (Crowley, 1962: 48). McCaffery (1972: 7-8) refers to nurses' response to the affective elements of the pain experience as the "psychological approach," as opposed to the physical and physiological approaches of physicians.

When pain cannot be alleviated, "the patient's needs for comforting and emotional support are increased a hundredfold; and the failure to give him this help because of one's own frustrations must be guarded against" (Crowley, 1962: 49). This emotional dedication, while certainly praiseworthy in this day of cold, instrumental relationships, can be a contraindication when applied to chronic pain. As we shall see below, clinical psychologists insist that "tender loving care" can inadvertently reinforce negative pain behaviors such as dependency and depression.

Nurses are at the forefront of the movement to provide special programs for pain-afflicted people. We must note, however, that the nurses who are taking the initiative in establishing a distinctively autonomous and nonmedical approach to chronic pain are among the relatively few nurses who are professionally oriented and seek functional autonomy from doctors. The vast majority of nurses adhere to traditionally bureaucratic work-role conceptions and do not commit themselves to the pursuit of long-range, professional career goals (Davis and Olesen, 1965). Nevertheless, nursing's involvement with chronic pain provides us with insight into the still-developing process of its professionalization.

The gate control theory provides a ready means for *scientifically* justifying a break with the dominant medical model of pain and pain management. Since nursing is essentially an applied rather than a theoretical science, it has been quite dependent upon the social and behavioral sciences for the conceptual frameworks upon which to base the "humanistic" facets of its work (Polit and Hunger, 1978: 76).[10] As a psychological conceptualization, the gate control theory is very conducive to nursing's traditional "holistic" approach to patient care. But equally important, the gate control theory provides a viable rationale for nonmedical pain modulation. Nursing's acknowledged proficiency in rehabilitation education, individualization of patient evaluation, and the administration of noninvasive treatments like biofeedback and transcutaneous electrical nerve stimulation fit the therapeutic regimens suggested by the gate control theory.

New roles have emerged to take advantage of this practical expertise. We now witness nurses acting as in-service and continuing education consultants on chronic pain management, sharing their knowledge with all sorts of health care workers.[11] Nurses' predispositions toward total pain patient care has helped them gain stature in the comprehensive/primary and holistic healing movements (Bauman, 1979: 47-53; Millis, 1977). Perhaps the most influential role gained to date is the executive administration of chronic pain centers (see Chapter 3). As Freidson (1970: 69) indicates, "To attain the autonomy of a profession, the paramedical occupation must control a fairly discrete area of work that be separated from the main body of medicine and that can be practiced *without routine contact with or dependence on medicine*" (italics added). Most chronic pain centers are either quasi-independent units within hospitals or totally independent facilities in which the physician is often limited to the role of *consultant* on medical matters (Resnick, 1977: 63-65). Nurses not only become equal partners in the "team" organization of many chronic pain centers, but as in the case of the pain unit attached to the Wilmington (Delaware) Medical Center, have applied their administrative acumen to the role of executive coordinator. As LeRoy (1977: 137) argues, "The nurse specialist is ideally suited to take leadership in [coordinating] an interested, experienced and compassionate team." As the concept of comprehensive chronic pain management spreads throughout the health care field, we can expect more nurses to take even greater initiative in defining its organizational and ideological parameters.

We should note that some nurses are influencing the direction of chronic pain care even while working within their traditional, organizational roles. Nurses have access to emerging information on chronic pain care through nursing publications, contact with other paramedical workers, and

continuing in-service training, which is required by law in
many states. This information not only shapes their own
work, but as several physicians have indicated to me, is
occasionally passed on informally to the doctor by means of
the "doctor/nurse game" described by Stein (1967). This
communication phenomenon, though obviously limited in
scope, exists as a result of nursing's somewhat close (closer
than medicine's) ties with other health care disciplines. For
example, several physicians have indicated that they have
learned from their nurses the benefits of prescribing low-
dosage analgesic drugs for chronic pain to be taken at regular
intervals.

Clinical Psychology

Attaching a single, meaningful definition to clinical psychology is an extremely difficult task. Although clinical psychologists have their own professional association and professional schools, their occupational goals and therapeutic
techniques differ. An adequate working definition is: *Clinical psychology is the application of psychological concepts
to the understanding and remediation of emotional, behavioral, and personality disorders through individual and
group therapy* (see also Wyatt, 1968: 222).[12] Garfield (1974:
15-18) notes three basic functions of clinical psychology:
(1) the administration and interpretation of diagnostic personality tests; (2) interactive psychotherapy; and (3) exploration through scientific research of basic processes of
normal and abnormal human behavior. The underlying motif
and *raison d'être* throughout clinical psychology's historical
development has been *problem solving,* as illustrated by its
evolution from what used to be commonly called abnormal
psychology in the early twentieth century (Garfield,
1965).[13]

In spite of clinical psychology's precarious identity, it
remains the most autonomous of the paramedical occupations. It is legally recognized as an independent profession in

most states and is self-governed through uniform, written ethical standards (Jacobs, 1976: 23; Freidson, 1970: 53-54). On the other hand, its dependence on medicine is largely determined by the fact that clinical psychologists cannot prescribe drugs, and that approximately 83 percent of the 23,000 registered clinical psychologists in the United States are employed in hospitals, clinics, and other medically controlled health care settings (Garfield, 1974: 441). There is a movement in the field, however, toward increased fee-for-service private practice, as clinical psychologists come to be identified more as health care workers than as mental health workers or diagnostic testers (Dorken and Whiting, 1974: 309; Schofield, 1975).

In contrast to nursing, clinical psychology has access to an independent if variegated body of scientific knowledge upon which to build an argument for professional status. Since theoretical psychology, like sociology, is a multiparadigmatic science, "clinical psychology has been the pawn of partisanship practically since its beginning" (Wyatt, 1968: 223). Psychoanalytic theory, modeling theory, the "self-theory" of Carl Rogers, association theory, and a host of other psychological frameworks have been used in measuring and treating personality disorders. There has recently been a resurgence of interest in *behavioral* conceptualizations (Bandura, 1974). This neobehavioralism is inspired less by Watson's classical notions of the conditioned reflex than by Skinner's (1969) theory of operant conditioning. In clinical form:

> Behavior therapy, as psychology in general, is going cognitive. . . . What the client says to himself (i.e., his appraisals, attributions, self-evaluations), or the self-statements and images that he emits prior to, accompanying, and following his overt behavior are becoming an increasingly important area for therapeutic intervention. . . . Behavior therapy is shifting in emphasis from a focus on discrete, situation-specific responses and problem-specific procedures to a

coping-skills model, which can be applied across situations and problems [Meichenbaum and Turk, 1976: 1-2].

This emphasis on the cognitive aspects of learning and behavior is compatible with one of the gate control theory's prime corollaries—namely, that both the *reaction to* and *perception of* pain is affected by cognitive activities such as culturally acquired predispositions, anxiety, attention, suggestion, and personal history of pain (Melzack and Dennis, 1978: 10). In this regard the gate control theory, itself of psychological origin, has merged with neobehavioralism to provide the theoretical basis for clinical psychology's entree into the field of chronic pain care.

The clinical psychological perspective on chronic pain is as follows. The medical differentiation between somatic and psychological pain is irrelevant, for the issue of whether or not a person's declaration of pain can be linked to (or caused by) actual tissue damage is secondary to the fact that pain from any cause is communicated through personality and behavioral displays. For incidents of chronic pain that defy medical diagnosis and/or treatment, clinical psychologists prefer the concept of *psychogenic pain*—that is, "pain which is better described and understood in psychological rather than physical language" (Sternbach, 1974: 21).[14] Although the actual experiences of acute and chronic, somatic and psychological pain are often quite similar, long-term psychogenic pain can have considerable deleterious effects on a person's mental health. In reverting, perhaps, to their roots in abnormal psychology, clinical psychologists view related pain behaviors in strictly pathological terms, for "the complaint of pain, by itself, is about as likely to be a sign of mental as of physical disorder" (Sternbach, 1974: 79). It should be noted that little or no attention is given to the possible positive aspects or effects of chronic pain behaviors on personal life adjustments, if for no other reason than theoretical closure.

Clinical studies, based almost exclusively on objective personality tests such as the Minnesota Multiphasic Personality Inventory (MMPI) and the Eysenck, show that chronic pain patients exhibit unusually high levels of emotional disturbance. Sternbach et al. (1973), for example, administered the MMPI to 117 low-back patients. Nineteen of them, considered "acute" cases because they had had pain for less than six months, fell within normal limits on all personality measures. The remaining 98, considered "chronic" because their pain was present for six months or longer, scored significantly high in hypochrondriasis, depression, and hysteria, the so-called "neurotic triad" (Sternbach, 1974: 16). Assuming that the chronic pain patients could have previously presented normal psychological profiles, the authors concluded that long-term concern with their pain problems resulted in emotional disturbance. Numerous other clinical studies have supported Sternbach et al.'s conclusion, in spite of growing criticism of the application of the MMPI to the analysis of chronic pain patients.[15]

The question remains whether the chronic pain patient is somehow predisposed to neurotic pain behavior or is the victim of the pain experience itself. The psychological and psychiatric literature provides arguments for both positions, but there appears to be consensus among clinical psychologists that *pain behavior is learned behavior* that becomes ingrained by means of both positive and negative reinforcement. Fordyce (1976: 29, 46-50) reviewed the literature on the relationship between childhood experiences and chronic pain behavior and found high correlation in various studies. The general argument is as follows. When children experience illness, they are also likely to experience some degree of threat to survival and/or body integrity. If childhood illness is frequent or of long duration, high anxiety levels will be reinforced. Children also learn depressive behaviors through physical punishment. The punished child experiences at least momentary concern for rejection and loss of love. The sense of alienation from parents is reinforced by the frequency and severity of the punishment, as well as by its accompanying pain. Unresolved tension between child and parent leads to repressed feelings of anxiety, depression, anger, guilt, and/or hostility. If these neurotic reactions to pain and suffering are firmly ingrained in the child's psyche, they may later emerge in the adult's response to chronic pain. Clinical researchers, again through the use of personality inventories, find that chronic pain patients tend to report childhoods more fraught with pain experiences and parental conflicts than do nonpain patients (Merskey and Spear, 1967; Pilling et al., 1967; Szasz, 1957).

Clinical psychologists also argue that neurotic pain behavior is learned and reinforced during and after the onset of adult pain. A patient may find that chronic pain has certain rewards, difficult to relinquish even after the physiological bases for the pain have diminished. Indeed, the rewards may be sufficient for the patient to display levels of pain far in excess of actual physical cause. The rewards or current reinforcement of pain behaviors come from the patient's family, disability compensation benefits, or even physicians themselves (Sternbach, 1974: 55-56; Fordyce, 1973: 123-128).

Take the woman, for example, who is married to a man who ordinarily gives her very little attention and affection. With the onset of severe low-back pain, her husband suddenly becomes very solicitous and caring. Since the pain succeeds in revitalizing her marriage, the woman has very little reason for getting well and relinquishing her dependency. As another example, we have the construction worker who hates the sweat and drudgery of his job. He may find that a work-related injury that results in disability compensation has related rewards for him: He can legitimately avoid work, and still maintain financial support for himself and his family. Again, the worker has very little incentive for getting well and trying to return to work, even if the pain vanishes.

The most popular mode of treatment in clinical psychology for chronic pain is behavioral modification (Fordyce, 1976: 74-99; Sternbach, 1974: 99-103; Davidson, 1976). Clinical psychologists argue that the more traditional psychodynamic approach to chronic pain—that is, the psychiatric perspective based on the disease model of illness—is ineffective in treating the emotional disorders associated with pain because it assumes that these disorders are caused by inherent personality pathologies. On the contrary, clinical psychologists maintain that neurotic pain behaviors (or operants) can develop in patients with any kind of personality makeup, so that the task at hand is to reinforce "well behaviors" (*correct* responses to pain), so that the patient can better cope with pain. Among behaviorist methods are the establishment of goal-directed behaviors by means of patient contracts, the systematic elimination of pain behavior reinforcers (attention given to the patient's condition, sympathy, and analgesic drug abuse), and the control of pain itself through cognitive therapies like biofeedback and hypnosis.

Clinical psychologists have been instrumental in the creation, administration, and staffing of many chronic pain centers. These units provide a clinical testing ground for psychological conceptualizations of and treatments for pain, operating under varying degrees of independence from the authority of the physician. In these settings the clinical psychologist can often be referred to as "Doctor" without feelings of self-consciousness and without having to look over one's shoulder to see if an "M.D." is lurking (see Sternbach, 1974: 3).

Medical Social Work

Of the three paramedical occupations we are reviewing, medical social work is undoubtedly the least autonomous and the most vaguely defined.[16] Medical social workers have not actively sought recognition as a distinct subspecialty, but instead have tied their professional aspirations to those of social workers in general (Denton, 1978: 217). Social work's claim to professional status has not, however, been very successful. Since social work's modern inception in the welfare reform programs of the Depression, social workers have practiced their art almost exclusively as employees of bureaucratic organizations and agencies, with little movement toward independent practice (Sobey, 1977: 10; Meyer, 1967: 399). For example, over two-thirds of the medical social workers in the United States are employed in the social work departments of hospitals. Only in recent years have social workers attempted to develop a "scientific" basis for their practice, and they still rely heavily on the social and behavioral sciences as conceptual and therapeutic resources (see Germain, 1973).

Social workers have always had difficulty convincing their audiences that their knowledge and skills are truly unique, since "there is no question that what social workers are employed to do is also done by less professionally trained persons" (Meyer, 1967: 394-395). A widely accepted stereotype of the social worker is that of a patient, "humanistic" person who can adequately fulfill the tedious bureaucratic task of completing innumerable reports and forms.[17] This somewhat accurate description often puts medical social workers in conflict with volunteer, indigenous, and auxiliary workers who view medical social workers as threats to their own work domains (Denton, 1978: 216). Medical social workers' identity crisis is compounded by the argument presented by other health workers that medical social workers do not provide direct health care to the patient, but deal only with the (less important) disruptive effects of illness on interpersonal and occupational relationships.

The medical social worker's niche in the comprehensive pain care *team* concept is, however, almost guaranteed by these extramedical considerations. In tune with growing concern over chronic pain's often disastrous impact on the *total* life of the patient, medical social workers have focused on solving family- and work-related problems. The detrimental effects of chronic pain on the family system are many:

> Sexual functioning is decreased; children are often required to assume care of the home; and the social activities of the family unit are curtailed. Family members are frustrated, angry and bitter, but are unusually unable to express these feelings initially because they feel that these responses to someone "in pain" would be unacceptable and cruel [Wyckoff, 1978: 159].

In addition, the patient's family often suffers from the *financial* burden of chronic pain, in terms of both lost income and sometimes catastrophic medical bills.

During the initial interview and assessment of patients entering the chronic pain center, the medical social worker tries to identify the life stresses occurring along with the onset of pain. Divorce, loss of employment, children leaving home, and other crises can weaken the patient's ability to cope with physical incapacity and discomfort. The anger and/or grief associated with these life changes may be inadvertantly redirected toward the medical profession for not effecting a cure (Wyckoff, 1978: 157-158). The medical social worker counsels the patient—by means of ego psychology, transactional analysis, social learning theory, or other modalities—to become aware of hidden frustrations and to learn how to cope with them openly and rationally. The medical social worker will then help other family members to learn how to express their feelings and develop constructive communication techniques with the patient and within the family circle (see Berkman, 1977: 93-94).

Since the majority of chronic pain center patients have experienced industrial injuries, the medical social worker often serves as liaison between the center and the disability cmpensation system that pays for the services. In conjunction with the occupational therapist (if one is available), the medical social worker implements retraining for those patients not able to return to their former jobs. In those chronic pain units attached to general hospitals, the medical social worker also serves as a liaison between the patient and available hospital and community support services—for instance, chapels, recreation rooms, transportation services, and nursing home care for elderly patients.

The gate control theory has only tangential relevance to the work of medical social workers. Their area of expertise lies in managing the life problems associated with being a patient and not in managing pain or pain behavior per se. In this regard one might say that the medical social worker acts as "patient advocate" in the midst of the organizational/governmental/educational complex with which the patient must contend in the search for health care meanings. Specialized psychological theories are relevant only to those few medical social workers who engage in behavioral therapy of some sort.

SUMMARY: TOWARD A SOCIOLOGY OF THE CHRONIC PAIN EXPERIENCE

The variable levels of professional status held by the four health care specialties we have reviewed provide a context for understanding their response to the chronic pain phenomenon. For medicine, chronic pain simply is an anomaly that poses little threat to its basic assumptions, a puzzle to be worked out in time according to the rules of the medical paradigm. Members of the paramedical occupations have taken advantage of medicine's therapeutic failure to propose alternative theoretical and interventionist strategies that supply the substance for claims of unique expertise and professional growth. In other words, the reality of chronic pain has been forced on medicine, while paramedical workers have openly and gladly appropriated it.

Medical and paramedical views of chronic pain, especially as they are presented in the literature cited in this chapter, but also as they appear in formal interviews, are necessarily incomplete. These statements are largely programmatic declarations of *how best to treat pain,* but they do not describe literally the actual everyday conduct of pain work. Furthermore, we must be skeptical of the image of the patient and the experience of pain implicitly and explicitly conveyed by these statements because of the inherent biases underlying their purpose.

The most pervasive bias is *ideological.* In the parlance of sociological functionalism, all occupational groups seeking either to establish or maintain a sense of identity must present a unified ideology to their markets in the outside world. This ideology serves two purposes: the establishment of occupational boundaries, which indicate that the services offered are unique, and the display of evidence that the particular occupation is best suited to perform the needed services (Taylor, 1968: 431-451; Goode, 1960: 902-904).[18] Programmatic statements on chronic pain are ideological to the degree that they furnish one-sided and thus oversimplified views of the pain experience. To assume that all pain-related behavior is psychologically pathological or to define chronic pain in strictly physiological terms is to ignore the immense complexity of the phenomenon. We should also be aware of the fact that while these occupational groups appear quite anxious to discuss each other's shortcomings, they downplay their own limitations.[19]

Medical and paramedical perceptions of the pain-afflicted person are filtered through a *clinical bias.* Health care workers ordinarily encounter the sufferer in the hospital, clinic, or office. In these settings, the subject is perceived either as a patient (when care is delivered) or as a client (when psychological evaluation or research is conducted). Although the social roles of patient and client are necessary to the accomplishment of health care delivery, they are only two of many social roles the subject occupies during the course of living with pain. Health care workers either ignore the everyday life of the patient/client as irrelevant to the therapeutic model in use or distort the integrity of this experience by seeking only indications of psychological, emotional, or social maladjustment. The clinical setting simply is not conducive to open and free communication with patients (Cicourel, 1964: 73-104).

A sociology of the chronic pain experience complements health care perspectives because it allows us to analyze *all* aspects of the coping process. Therefore, we will *bracket* or *suspend* belief in the facticity of health care perspectives in order to view chronic pain through the perspective of the sufferer (see Schultz, 1970: 275-276). This is not to say that the perceptions of health care workers are necessarily wrong or of no objective use; they are simply incomplete. It is especially important to suspend belief in the view the people with pain are necessarily psychologically pathological. Without making this moral judgment, we can analyze them simply as people of common sense seeking meaning for their experience of embodied distress.

NOTES

1. The development of Western health care theory and practice is well documented by medical historians. Walker (1954) is among the best general histories of medicine. For a clear exposition of the relationship of medical progress to other changes in modern society, see McKeown (1965). Shryock's (1960) book is recognized by most historians as the best introduction to American medicine. Leavitt and Numbers (1978) provide an interesting collection of essays on specific medical and public health practices in America.

2. See Jakobovitz (1967) for a discussion of Old Testament/Jewish attitudes toward illness. See Lewis (1961) for a classic statement of New Testament/Christian attitudes toward pain and suffering.

3. Descartes's lectures on physiology can be found in the sections on *L'Homme* in "The Philosophical Works" (1955).

4. Sinclair (1967) reviews the various extensions and refinements of Von Frey's theory. Interestingly, there is still much debate among specificity theorists over the location of the pain center in the brain that supposedly interprets pain impulses automatically (see Melzack, 1973: 132).

5. Sternback (1968: 130-131) suggests that psychotherapy and electroshock therapy are among the few successful treatments for phantom limb pain.

6. The historical practice of applying electrical stimulation to painful areas may also be effective in closing the gate (Wooden, 1977). Shealy (1974b) and others

have applied this notion to the use of transcutaneous electrical stimulation of peripheral nerves associated with chronic pain syndrones.

7. Illich (1976) and Dubos (1959), on the contrary, are among the most vocal critics of medical claims of controlling infectious disease. Illich argues that the public health movement has been most instrumental in alleviating the social and cultural bases for disease. Dubos agrees with this position, but goes on to argue that infectious diseases of the truly epidemic variety appear to have natural cycles *independent* of medical intervention.

8. Rapid technological advancement and the growth of the modern hospital as a complex organization have led to the establishment of numerous "allied" health occupations. While laboratory, x-ray, physiotherapy, and other types of technicians do perform services related to chronic pain patients, they have much too little control over their work to have much say in the *design* of chronic pain care. Instead of actively seeking independent, professional status, they seek assimilation into what one spokesman projects to be the "one greater health profession" (Pellegrino, 1977: 32).

9. For a historical analysis of the emergence of modern nursing, see Bullough and Bullough (1965). Davis (1966) provides a distinctively sociological appraisal of nursing.

10. In fact, many professionally oriented nurses still seek doctoral training in the social sciences in spite of the new Ph.D. and D.N. degree programs being established in nursing. This trend is especially prevalent among those nurses who desire to do research on an academic level (see Cleland, 1976; Lenburg, 1975).

11. The services of nurse consultants are being made increasingly available through nonprofit, continuing education programs such as the Dee Evers and Associates group in San Diego, California. This particular program offers in-service courses required of registered nurses by the California Board of Registered Nursing.

12. Kelly (1966) represents the view of some clinical psychologists that their occupation should not be constrained by one dogmatic definition of purpose, especially during this period of transition and plurality of interests.

13. There has been intense competition between clinical psychology and psychiatry over the right to treat mental illness. Psychiatrists, on the one hand, argue that psychotherapy is a form of medical treatment that they alone, as M.D.s, should utilize. Clinical psychologists, on the other hand, argue that many types of emotional and behavioral disturbance without organic bases are better conceptualized and treated in ways differing from the medical model. Regardless of the effectiveness of treatment, psychiatrists maintain higher status and prestige as a group because of their professional ties with medicine (see Garfield, 1974: 18-24).

14. This differs from the more traditional, *medical* definition of psychogenic pain as that which has psychological rather than physical *causes* (Fordyce, 1976: 26-29).

15. Wolff (1977: 47) argues that:

We have factor analyzed the MMPI and have not been able to demonstrate any statistically significant relationships between the resultant MMPI factors and pain variables. On the other hand, Sternbach . . . has been, and apparently still is, using the MMPI as a tool for analyzing pain. In my opinion, his interpretations are somewhat open to criticism, as he utilizes small changes or nuances in responses within the normal range, which were never intended to be interpreted in this manner and lack solid statistical support.

16. For a general overview of the field of social work, see Fink (1974). An interesting collection of essays on recent developments in medical social work can be found in Bracht (1978).

17. As is the case with most stereotypes, there is an element of truth in the image of the social worker as do-gooder. Rosenberg (1957), for example, found that social workers as a group are highly service oriented, much more so than, say, physicians.

18. In this regard, we can say that the image of an occupation—constructed through reports, policy statements, and programatic declarations—is a form of bureaucratic propaganda. Altheide and Johnson (1979: 2) define bureaucratic propaganda as "any report produced by an organization for evaluation and other practical purposes, which is targeted for individuals, committees, or publics that are unaware of its promotive character and the editing processes that shaped the report."

19. The recent emergence of the specialty of behavioral medicine is an example of efforts to create a unified and legitimate identity for psychologists working in the medical system. Pinkerton et al. (1982: 3) define behavioral medicine as "the clinical application of principles, techniques, and procedures of behavior therapy in the assessment, treatment, management, rehabilitation, and prevention of physical disease or concomitant behavioral reactions to physical dysfunction." Although the term "behavioral medicine" is new, this specialty incorporates a range of existing psychological modalities such as operant conditioning, biofeedback, and relaxation training.

3

BECOMING A
PAIN-AFFLICTED PERSON

I practice good medicine on good people and bad medicine on bad people.

> —*Sam Two Feathers, medicine man, explaining why he cast a fatal spell on an enemy*

To define an individual as a pain-afflicted person is to account for the past, present, and future status of the problem. The term "chronic" is fairly vague in meaning, but occupational physicians and disability insurance workers officially consider pain to be chronic when it lasts for more than six months (Finneson, 1977: 37-43). We ordinarily conceive of chronic pain as an adult affliction. Physicians rarely talk about childhood chronic pain because of the predominance of acute illness among children. As one physician notes, "Children don't have chronic pain. They either quickly recover or they die" (quoted in Neal, 1978: 139).[1] Like other types of chronic illness, chronic pain is most often associated with the aging process, but unlike other types of chronic illness, chronic pain is not limited to the elderly. Spinal problems, migraine headaches, and arthritis can strike people of all ages.

Chronic pain is not an immediately discernible disease. While an individual can be diagnosed as a diabetic simply on the basis of routine laboratory tests, a diagnosis of chronic pain comes only after an arduous process of finding out that the pain is not transitory and will not heal in the ordinary sense of the word. Thus it is useful to conceive of the process of *becoming* a chronically pain-afflicted person as a "career" (Freidson, 1970: 242-243; Roth, 1963) marked by certain sequential events and experiences that culminate in a definition of the pain as a disease and not simply symptomatic of disease.

The essential argument of this chapter is that there are two contrasting themes in the emergence of a chronic pain career: *clinical* and *experiential.* Clinically, the medical evaluation of a pain condition progresses linearly from acute to chronic designation. Medical workers initially react to pain as transitory, and it is only after long and repeated therapeutic failure that a negative prognosis is given. In other words, chronic pain is pain that is medically unsuppressable. Experientially, the path of the career is most notably marked by a situationally effective struggle to maintain a sense of control over one's pain. This control refers not only to the alleviation (if not the elimination) of pain, but also the maintenance of both personal bodily integrity and the presentation of a competent self, which the pain experience tends to destroy. The normal chronic pain career is interspersed with episodes during which the person loses control of pain. Suffering can then become a meaningless experience that leads to hopelessness, anger, and other negative feelings. Tension between these two career themes can lead to conflict between the patient and the health care worker because pain-afflicted people commonly reject the clinical designation of inevitability and adhere to the belief (and hope) that the pain will somehow be eliminated in the future.

There are three major stages in the chronic pain career. The first stage involves the onset of pain. An individual reacts to pain in much the same way he or she reacts to any apparently acute health problem, that is, by attempting self-help and then entering the normal and appropriate channels of professional health care. The second stage begins when conservative treatments fail and more radical interventions are attempted (e.g., surgery). The third stage reflects the awareness of the failure of all medical interventions, the medical designation of chronicity, and the patient's search for alternative forms of help. Throughout these three stages, the impact of the family is critical. Family members' flexibility in accepting or rejecting the often lengthy and costly search for a cure is especially important.

I base my detailed discussion of these three stages on the experience of back pain, the most common form of intense chronic pain. When the career contingencies of other sources of chronic pain differ meaningfully, they will be duly noted.[2] The most important difference is that treatment of chronic back pain more commonly results in surgery, especially if the etiology is thought to be intervertabral disc degeneration (i.e., slipped disc). Most other forms of chronic pain rarely result in surgical intervention.

I have decided to portray the process of becoming a pain-afflicted person in one, fairly unitary career model, rather than constructing several models to indicate possible social, economic, or cultural variation. There are two justifications for this approach. First, the pain biographies I elicited during my research were very similar. Pain-afflicted people in general face the same health care decisions and feel the same emotional responses regardless of station in life. Second, I feel strongly that my study has arrived at the *essence* of the chronic pain experience. Due to the exploratory nature of this study, it seems wise to describe as elegantly as possible the transcendent elements of the chronic pain experience and to understand them well before proposing further research to explore relevant SEC variations.

STAGE I: THE ONSET OF PAIN

One would not be human if one did not know and experience pain. Our lives are circumscribed by pain, for life begins and ends under the shroud of physical suffering. Everyday life is interspersed with episodes of varying discomfort ranging from the cuts and bruises that accompany childhood adventures to all too common after-the-party hangovers. Since everyday pain is such a common and transitory experience, we usually manage to cope with it by uttering an impulsive expletive, rubbing our wounds, taking a few aspirin, and accepting it all as a natural part of living. Our concern intensifies, however, when pain is severe, unremitting, or associated with a serious injury. We then seek help from healers whom we perceive as qualified to eliminate both the pain and its underlying cause.[3]

Chronic pain begins much like other types of pain. We should note, however, that a definite age factor influences the initial meaning of chronic pain. Chronic pain is commonly associated with a traumatic injury for young adults, with developmental problems like arthritis the exception. Young adults assume that, in light of their youth and overall good health, even the most severe pain will either go away through natural healing or through regular medical intervention. Mark is a 24-year-old construction worker with a three-year history of lower back pain eminating from a work-related injury. At first, he justifiably defined his pain as acute and nonproblematic:

When the ladder slipped and I fell, I landed flat on my back. It hurt like hell and I knew I probably broke something. . . . I really didn't expect to be out of work all that long. A lot of guys are always getting hurt on the job and shaking it off. I figured that the doc would fix me up quick. . . . I play a lot of sports and always get banged up. I figured I would be able to get over this back thing just like everything else.

For the older person who is less active and therefore less prone to traumatic injury, the initial episode of pain is commonly associated with the contingencies of aging. The pain associated with degenerative diseases such as cancer, arthritis, and *tic douloureux* are routinely defined at the onset as chronic by the pain person. Since it fits the overall experience of growing old, ongoing pain is considerably less traumatic and problematic for the elderly. Martha is an 81-year-old widow with trigeminal neuralgia that results in extreme facial pain:

I don't think of it as a sickness . . . just a malady that you can't shake, like hay fever. . . . A friend used to call everyday and ask "Is your face hurting right now?" Of course it hurt, so I told her to stop asking. When you get old I guess there's not much else to do but talk about your illnesses.

Age-specific responses to initial episodes of pain are, of course, variable from situation to situation. Some young adults who are normally quite anxious about illness symptoms can be alarmed by pain; some older people who have never been seriously ill can be devastated by unexplainable pain. The point is that young adults find it very difficult to entertain the thought of suffering pain for the rest of their lives.

When nontraumatic pain first occurs, a person attempts to make sense of it through personal reflection on past experience with pain. One may define back pain as minor and transitory because previous episodes of back pain or backache seemed to go away pretty much by themselves. Migraine headaches are initially "normalized" in much the same way, as the following example illustrates. Mr. Franklin is a middle-aged business executive whom I met one afternoon in a chiropractor's office. He began experiencing piercing headaches approximately a year earlier. At first, Mr. Franklin assumed that he could treat these headaches with aspirin just as he had done for years:

> Ever since I finished law school and entered business, sure, I got an occasional headache or two. You know, job pressures, deadlines, and all that. So when the migraines started, I didn't think much of it. I figured that a few aspirins and a day or two out of the office would suffice.

Mr. Franklin's previous experience with headaches betrayed him for, although they presented symptoms that were somewhat similar to the current pain, he was later to learn that his migraine headaches are based upon a constriction of the intercranial arteries and not simple work-related tension.[4]

One may also reflect on the pain experiences of others. One's own symptoms can be compared with another person's similar symptoms, assuming that the prognosis will be the same. This type of comparison can also be quite deceiving. Marsha is a 26-year-old mother and housewife. During her first pregnancy, she felt moderate soreness in the small of her back. In trying to make sense of the pain, she remembered her mother once mentioned that she too suffered backaches during pregnancy which she felt were caused by the added burden of carrying a child. Marsha assumed that her pain had a similar cause; however, several months after giving birth she consulted an orthopedic physician and learned that the pain was really caused by a degenerated lumbar disc.

When an individual's personal reflection fails to make sense of nontraumatic pain, family members or friends are consulted. This network of available, significant others provides two services. First, they can help the pain person evaluate the *nature* of the problem. This assistance is crucial for the individual because spontaneous pain is difficult to define alone. For example, a ruptured or "slipped" lumbar disc usually results in the sensation of sharp pain radiating down one leg. One's first reaction is to try to locate the problem in the leg itself. The experience of sciatic pain, in itself, gives little indication that the problem originates in the spinal area. Unless one has extensive medical knowledge, this information must be obtained from others.[5]

Second, significant others provide what Freidson (1970: 290-297) refers to as a "lay referral system." When the pain is perceived as being sufficiently serious to warrant medical help, the individual usually learns of medical options from friends and family members. Freidson's differentiation between "parochial" and "cosmopolitan" relations between lay persons and health care professionals is relevant to chronic pain:

> The lower-class system in the United States might be called parochial both because of the limitations of its culture and the limitation of its organized connections with the medical institutions. Neither lower-class patients nor their lay consultants are very familiar with the range of medical services available. . . . In contrast to the lower-class, the middle-class patient participates in what I have called a cosmopolitan sytem. First of all, he needs less help from others. Markedly more prone to make decisions about medical care without the aid of lay consultants outside the household, more familiar with abstract criteria for professional qualifications, better acquainted with a number of professional practices if only by his residential mobility, and more knowledgeable about illness itself, he is likely to feel more secure in his own diagnosis and his own assessment of the virtures of the care he receives [Freidson, 1970: 290-291].

In the case of both the lower and middle class, pain-afflicted people consult healers in accord with their perceptions of available options. Members of the lower class are normally channeled through public or quasi-public clinics, while members of the middle class normally consult their family physicians just as they would for any kind of illness. The knowledgeable "cosmopolitan" person may even go directly to a specialist for help.

The working-class person, however, presents a unique situation not accounted for by Freidson (1970), Mechanic (1978: 132-157), Suchman (1965a, 1965b), and other students of the physician/patient encounter. Working-class persons are more liable to incur job-related injuries than members of other social classes (see Finneson, 1977: 38). When pain emerges from a job-related injury, the lay referral system is of little use because the employee may have little choice but to consult the company physician or nurse. Traumatic injury in general presents few options because it is normally treated as an emergency situation, with the potentially pain-afflicted person largely dependent on immediate others to call an ambulance (which is probably under orders to take all clients to the nearest emergency facility) or to personally arrange for expedient health care.

The recent development of *comprehensive health care* is also a factor, though a minor one at this point in time, in lessening the importance of the lay referral system. A comprehensive health care unit provides all health care services required by its members (see Burns, 1973). Its members no longer need to "shop around" for services as happens when people are dependent upon fee-for-service health care. Thus the pain-afflicted person normally consults his or her health care team automatically.

We should note, however, that many cases of pain never arrive at the stage of physician consultation. A relatively small proportion of pain-afflicted people immediately consult chiropractors, naturapaths, and other nonmedical healers.[6] This avoidance of medicine occurs only when an individual's subcultural influences present nonmedical healing as a "normal" course of action for virtually any illness, as is common among some sectors of the rural population (see McCorkle, 1961; see also Chapter 4). Self-treatment is used when the person perceives the discomfort as a natural result of his or her station in life. The best example of this is the "bad back" phenomenon, so common among manual laborers. A person who works hard for a living comes to expect aches and pains. Among manual laborers in the railroad industry, "railroad back" is a common ailment. This condition is indicated by a hunching of and a lack of mobility in the back. Railroad workers think little of back pain because they expect it from the extensive stooping and lifting which are part of the job. One old timer told me:

> Oh, yah, I'd sit in a hot tub everyday after coming home from the yard. . . . I guess I was lucky that my ole lady was good at rubbing me down. . . . All the fellas working the yard just hoped that their backs would hold out until they could retire.

(Later in this chapter, I will discuss *spondylitis,* an arthritic condition that may be genetic yet controllable by means of anti-inflammatory drugs. Many cases of railroad back may in fact be spondylitis; see Fisk, 1977: 56.) Koos (1954) indicated in his now classic study of health care in a midsized city that although lower back pain is a common condition among lower- and working-class women, it is not considered by them to be symptomatic of any specific disease or disorder, but simply part of their everyday existence.

When the individual first encounters medicine, the primary goal is the achievement of *control* over the pain through diagnosis and treatment. Control is passed on to the physician because of trust in his or her expertise. This trusting dependence leads to open and objective presentation of symptoms. *Many pain-afflicted people first consult physi-*

*cians in order to verify their belief that the pain is simple
and transitory.*

Physicians routinely diagnose pain as "real" and as having a physiological basis, leading to conservative treatment.[7] Back pain may be attributed to minor muscle strain that calls for conservative treatment like bed rest, heat application, and mild analgesics. From the physician's perspective, it is best to begin with conservative interventions, because the severity of the problem is unknown, and then progress to more radical treatments as needed. The pain-afflicted person, on the contrary, perceives the physician's conservative stance as *definitive,* so that ineffective treatment may lead to discreditation of the physician's expertise:

> Dr. Stuart kept telling me that my backache would go away in time if I learned to take it easy and quit burning the candle at both ends. I had a feeling that the problem was more serious than that but, you know, the doctor knows best. I don't think he really realized how bad the pain was, but that's his job to find out.

This patient echoes the common complaint that physicians tend to underestimate the severity of suffering. However, most patients do not realize that they present symptoms very objectively and tend themselves to refrain from describing the true level of discomfort. Underlying this stoic presentation of self is a feeling that physicians are too busy and too professional to want to hear complaints. This feeling may be largely derived from previous experience with physicians or from a sense of self-conscious awe in which the physician is held.

STAGE II: THE EMERGENCE OF DOUBT

As the pain persists and conservative diagnosis and treatment continue to be ineffective, the patient is normally referred to a specialist for further consultation. This can be either the physician's or the patient's decision, depending on who first concludes that the conservative treatment has been ineffective. The criteria for making this decision, however, are defined by the pain person, who is the only one able to tell whether or not the pain has lessened. For back pain patients, referral is made either to an orthopedic or a neurological physician/surgeon.[8] An orthopedic physician is consulted when the problem is believed to be mechanical, such as a degenerated disc, whereas a neurologist is consulted when specific nerve pathology is suspected (e.g., neuralgia). The choice is not always so objective. The physician may simply refer his or her patient to whomever is known in the community to be a "good back person" regardless of specialization.

Although the individual is somewhat disappointed that the family physician did not help much, a feeling of security accompanies the referral. By this time, the pain-afflicted person realizes that the problem is not transitory, so that the specialist's complex-sounding diagnosis is comfortably reassuring:

I'm sure that Dr. Thorpe [the family physician] did all he could for me. . . . When he told me that there might be nerve damage, and that I should probably see a back specialist, I told him to find me the best in town. Williams [a neurologist] was supposedly the best around, so I immediately made an appointment to see him. . . . I thought that if he couldn't help me, who could? . . . I really felt great when he said that I had a bulging disc in the lumbar area. At least now they could *do* something, you know what I mean?

The pain person's control of the situation is maintained as responsibility is transferred from the general practitioner/ family physician to the specialist. The prestige of the specialist also helps the pain person to maintain control of the presentation of the pain to others. One of the prime requisites in displaying *competence* to others in interaction is to show that *one has wisely sought the best available health care.* Although the pain person may privately entertain doubts about the specialist's effectiveness, the specialist's qualifications and reputation are discussed with others in only the most complimentary terms. To do otherwise would reduce the legitimacy of complaining about the suffering incurred. By giving the impression that one is not coping with the illness properly, the pain person is liable to discrediting evaluations by others (e.g., "it serves you right," or "it's your own fault for trying to save a little money").

The specialist may prescribe either additional conservative treatment or hospitalization, first for further testing and then for radical intervention if necessary. Hospitalization is an ironic experience for these individuals because they undergo diagnostic and therapeutic procedures that in themselves are sometimes more painful than the original experience of pain. Fagerhaugh and Strauss (1977: 85) have noted the irony of *inflicted pain:*

> One of the often unrecognized ironies attending the work of health personnel is that they who minister to pain may inflict pain. Indeed, this may be a fairly inevitable part of their jobs. A considerable proportion of work with and around patients involves the inflicting of pain. It is associated, of course, with a host of essential tasks: with diagnosis, surgery, various therapies, regimens, and even with the mechanics of giving adequate nursing care. Most of such induced pain is necessary although some of it is surely not.

Furthermore, Fagerhaugh and Strauss argue that patients and staff negotiate an implicit contract by which the patient agrees to endure inflicted pain with a minimum of disruptive pain expression and the staff agrees to minimize the intensity and duration of inflicted pain. Conflict arises when either party fails to live up to these perceived expectations. Pain-afflicted people also negotiate control over inflicted pain, but the net result is more emotionally devastating than it is for the average acute patient. From the pain-afflicted person's perspective, ongoing pain is the essential reason for hospitalization. It is much more than simply an unpleasant by-product of hospitalization. Pain-afflicted people in general find it quite difficult to understand why they should be expected to endure any more pain. They may respond to any additional pain by not only questioning the competency and humanity of the staff, but also by beginning to question the entire medical ethos.

The two most prevalent clinical procedures that inflict great pain on patients with spinal conditions are *myelography* and *traction*.[9] Myelography is a diagnostic procedure in which a metallic dye is injected into the spinal canal to allow certain pathologies to be visible on x-ray film (LeRoy, 1977: 180). The neurological staff rarely prepare patients for this extreme pain and understate the procedure's inaccuracy and potential dangers:

> When my doctor told me to have a myelogram, he said it was just for x-rays, and you know that they don't hurt. . . . The myelogram was the worst thing I ever did. It hurt like hell when they stuck that knitting needle in my back. On top of everything, I couldn't believe that they couldn't agree on what disc was slipped on the TV monitor. I'm sure they just finally guessed.

The above patient suffered intense headaches for several days after the myelogram was performed. The physician did warn him that some of the dye might possibly remain in the spinal canal afterwards and that excessive movement in bed might cause the dye to enter the brain. This warning, however, was nullified by the ward nurse's apparently incorrect advice that there was very little chance of negative side effects.[10]

Traction is a therapeutic procedure that is used to relieve muscle spasms by means of stretching the spinal column (Fisk, 1977: 134-135). Although physicians consider traction to be a conservative treatment, it can be extremely painful. The pain is magnified subjectively by the fact that a person may be placed in traction for hours or even days on end while finding very little relief from the original pain (see also Wiener, 1975: 510).[11]

When the patient realizes that these painful procedures are ineffective, emerging skepticism of the powers of medicine is often matched with a plunge into deep depression. Some (although relatively few according to health care workers) patients actually entertain thoughts of suicide. Suicide is a crucial problem in orthopedic wards, where the level of inflicted pain is especially high. As would be expected, hospital administrators try to mask the reality of clinical suicide from critical observation. The orthopedic ward in one general hospital, for example, is on the sixth floor and architecturally designed, like the rest of the hospital, with waist-high windows that open to the outside. One of the male orderlies describes the opportunities this situation presents to depress pain-afflicted patients:

> Since I've been working there [three years], two patients have actually committed suicide. From what I hear, a whole lot of others have tried. . . . One old guy just wheeled himself up to the window, opened it up, and pushed himself out. The honchos [administrators] got wise and sealed all the windows, like they had to do in the psychiatric ward.

According to several workers in this hospital, pain-related suicides are officially accounted for by blaming the patient for having inherent psychopathological tendencies prior to admission to the hospital. The issue of locating cause for clinical suicide is clouded by the fact that inflicted pain and the original pain are confounded by both the patient and the staff, so it is analytically quite difficult to state which type of pain is unbearable. Suicidal tendencies probably result from a combination of both.[12]

Throughout the initial period of hospitalization, the average patient experiences a sense of embarrassment for "not really being sick" but taking up the time and space needed for sick people with really critical problems. Ongoing pain is usually defined more as a condition than as an *illness* because the patients perceive their problems as something that is to be fixed rather than healed. For example, many patients often question the necessity of daily blood tests, injections, and the like, which they feel are only relevant to patients with infectious diseases. The switch from the definition of condition to the definition of illness comes only when surgery or other radical interventions are ordered.[13]

The attending physician prescribes surgery for back patients when it appears that the pain is caused by severe disc degeneration, congenital malfunctioning of the spinal area, and so on. The patient's decision about whether or not to undergo surgery is, however, problematic. If the physician's diagnosis is contrary to the commonsense experience of pain, the patient may balk. For example, a patient may disvalue the physician's diagnosis that radiating leg pain is caused by a ruptured lumbar disc, especially if the patient feels no pain in the lumbar region of the back. Experientially, it is absurd to argue that the cause of pain can be so far removed from the actual location of pain. The patient may refuse surgery if the physician's explanation of the problem is unclear or if the patient has less than total trust in the physician's judgment.

A more common reaction to the suggestion of surgery is based on a fear of surgery in general. Surgery is readily perceived as a fundamental threat to bodily integrity. One factor producing this fear is the experience of embodiment:

> I just can't imagine letting some knife-happy doctor cut open my back. I mean, your back is like the, uh, foundation of your body. It doesn't have many parts of its own, but supports all the other parts, like your heart or liver. . . . Just think about it. If your back gets ruined, you can't walk, you can't lift anything, and you can't [have sexual intercourse].

We all have a sense of the fragility of the body. We protect our bodies from unnecessary intrusion, whether it is well intended or not. Suffering patients often resort to folklore to support existentially based anxieties:

> Dr. Phillips told me that all the tests showed a ruptured disc. . . . I really freaked out. My folks warned me that back surgery is really dangerous. My father's friend at work has to wear a back brace for the rest of his life because he says his doctor screwed up. . . . You wouldn't believe how many people are paralyzed from bad back operations.

When I asked the above patient for the source of her information on the large numbers of surgically produced paralytics, she simply said that she heard it someplace. From the medical perspective, however, there is little risk involved with back surgery beyond the normal risks associated with any surgery (e.g., anesthesia and postoperative complications).

But there is a situational factor that influences the decision-making process, regardless of any transcendent feelings towards one's body or surgery in general. If the physician recommends surgery immediately after diagnostic testing while the patient is still in the hospital, the tendency is for the patient to consent immediately. There are two reasons why this happens. First, the physician convincingly argues that they should proceed with the surgery because the patient is already in the hospital; this saves both the physician and the patient the inconvenience of having to be readmitted at a later date. Second, the medical setting itself leaves many patients feeling quite powerless in opposing the physician's will. The notion that pervades the patient/staff interaction is that the patient is there to be helped and, if surgery is required, the patient has given at least *implicit* consent to the staff to do what is best for the patient. If the physician recommends surgery after the patient has been discharged from the hospital, the patient can more easily forestall it.

By making his or her decision outside of the hospital setting, the patient is free to both reflect on the pros and cons of
surgery and consult the lay referral system for advice. Needless to say, commonsense arguments against the advisability
of surgery are more powerful outside of the hospital, for surgery within the hospital is a routine, everyday procedure. In
other words, the patient can be talked out of surgery by peers
as easily as he or she can be talked into surgery by health care
workers.[14]
Nevertheless, few patients actually refuse their first pain
surgeries. Trust in medicine, although probably diminished
to some degree by the ineffectiveness of medicine in the past,
is usually sufficiently strong to warrant compliance with the
physician's wishes. Patients place high expectations on the
wisdom of the physician, so that in the absence of convincing
arguments from the lay sector against surgery, they more or
less *drift* into the operating room situation. Patients enter
surgery with the understanding that the *real* cause of the pain
will be eliminated. They are rarely told that *only 30 percent
or so of all laminectomies* (i.e., disc operations) *are reasonably effective* (see Shealy, 1974a), although they are reassured that the risks of complications from the much-feared
"slip of the knife that ends with paralysis" are minimal. The
pain patient thus enters the operating room with the highest
expectations of serious albeit routine surgical procedures
that are almost always officially reported as "successful"
and "uneventful" at their conclusion.[15]

STAGE III: THE CHRONIC PAIN EXPERIENCE

For some sufferers, surgery marks the end of their long
ordeal. Their pain never comes to be defined as chronic,
although these patients are commonly warned by their
physicians never to place excessive strain on their backs in
order to avoid reinjury. But for those patients whose pain

continues, the failure of surgery is not immediately discernible. They feel very little pain after surgery because of the aftereffects of massive anesthesia. As the effects of the anesthesia wear off, what might be perceived as the original pain may gradually return. The attending physician normalizes this pain by defining it as routine "postoperative pain" that will eventually diminish as the surgical lesions heal.[16]

After discharge from the hospital, the attending physician advises the pain person to adhere closely to an exercise regimen that is intended to strengthen the back muscles. Remarkably, these prescribed exercises are rarely followed. Stressful rehabilitative exercises like the Williams schedule are very painful in themselves. Pain persons shy away from this self-inflicted discomfort because it reminds too much of the original pain:

> I really didn't want to disobey the doctor, but I didn't have the heart to endure any more suffering. I just wanted to be comfortable for a change.

This fear of additional pain is often matched by a *fear of reinjury* due to stressful exercise. Back patients are especially careful to not take the chance of foolishly hurting themselves and putting themselves through the nightmare of pain again. Experientially, the choice of allowing the lesion to properly heal makes more sense than the physician's admonition that the lesion will heal properly only with rigorous exercise.[17] But patients are not likely to tell their physicians that they are not keeping up with the exercises for fear of appearing to be incompetent. This evasion and/or lying may mark the beginning of constrained communication between the physician and the patient.

The postoperative period also marks the genesis of analgesic drug abuse for many pain persons. Large dosages of painkillers are administered to the postoperative patient for surgically related pain that is thought to be simple and transitory. As the so-called postoperative pain lingers and becomes confounded with the return of the original pain, the pain person may have already become dependent on the drugs to maintain belief in the effectiveness of surgery. A similar state of confusion exists in the early career of the person whose chronic pain turns out to be surgically iatrogenic (Illich, 1976: 134-135). Margaret is a 46-year-old housewife who was hospitalized for a digestive disorder. Her surgery solved the digestive problem conclusively, but the pain due to multiple incisions in the viscera has lasted unabated for five years. Margaret began taking large dosages of Demerol right after surgery and continued to do so as the pain lasted. I talked to Margaret as she was waiting for an appointment to see the director of a local pain clinic from whom she hoped to get help in controlling her drug habit:

> My doctor did warn we that the recuperation would be long and painful. Nine, ten Demerol a day, but no big deal. . . . We figured that I wouldn't need the pills for long but, boy were we wrong! . . . I still can't even get out of bed in the morning without my "helpers."

Margaret estimates that she has taken an average of twelve Demerols or Percodans a day. This dosage is not, however, unusually high for chronic pain sufferers (see Lennard et al., 1971: 1-15). Drug abuse problems of chronic arthritic patients take a different form. They may be treated with anti-inflammatory agents (e.g., steroids and cortisone) which, if continued over a long period of time, can lead to gastric ulceration and weakness in the joints (Sergeant, 1969: 132; Bonica, 1953: 1123-1126).[18]

As the surgery fades into the past but the pain persists, we witness the emergence of patient independence. The pain-afflicted person no longer places blind trust in the physician, for medical ineffectiveness often results in distinct feelings of betrayal. Specific patient demands such as new treat-

ments, different kinds of drugs, and referrals to other specialists now replace open-ended requests for help based upon
the physician's better judgment. Knowledge of these medical alternatives is obtained through the return to the lay
referral system. As pain-afflicted people become more and
more obsessed with their problem, they become increasingly
sensitized to the experience and advice of others who have
had similar problems and may have access to different kinds
of help. In this regard, we could say that there is a *chronic
pain subculture* that exists to disseminate information and
to offer comfort to its members. The pain-afflicted person
gains a sense of camaraderie from knowing that he or she is
not alone or unique in coping with chronic pain. Theresa, a
26-year-old back patient, became involved with the chronic
pain subculture while talking to other patients in her physician's waiting room.

> It's amazing how many people you run across who've been
> screwed over by doctors, too. . . . I first met Fran in the wait-
> ing room. She told me about this acupuncturist in Seaview
> who was helping her more than the doctor was, needless to
> say. . . . I got involved with a bunch who go to all the pain
> talks [seminars]. It's really great because we understand
> what each other is going through.

Besides the physician's office, other sources of contact with
the chronic pain subculture include family members, neigh-
bors, friends, the media, and even chance encounters with
strangers. (In Chapters 5 and 6 I will discuss the importance
of the chronic pain subculture to specific occupationally
related pain problems.)

A chronic pain career can get totally out of control if the
person maintains unrealistic hope in the ultimate power of
medicine. A common rationale for this position is something
like the following: "Somewhere there is a doctor who can
help me. It's just a matter of time, patience, and locating

him." At worst, this hope translates into repeated surgeries that are rarely effective for back patients (see also Pace, 1976: 115-116). Subsequent surgeries may include spinal fusions and rhizotomies (Williams, 1978).[19] There are back patients who have undergone up to twenty unsuccessful surgeries. Such irrational behavior can only be accounted for the fact that, in general, pain-afflicted people reject the label "chronic" because they refuse to believe that they must be in pain for the rest of their lives.

CONNING THE PHYSICIAN

As pain-afflicted people begin searching out other health care practitioners, including nonmedical practitioners (see Chapter 4), they engage in what is commonly referred to as "doctor hopping" (Pace, 1976: 54-59; Sternbach, 1974: 68-77). Disgruntled physicians argue that veteran patients shop around for health care services more to confound, test, and "get even" with physicians than to actually get help. From the patient's perspective, real help is being sought, but the presentation of symptoms must be guarded and managed in light of changes in physicians' definitions of the problem, according to the following process. When physicians decide that they can no longer help the person, they label the problem "chronic" pain. The diagnostic focus shifts from the pain per se to problems faced in coping with the pain. The label "chronic pain person" implicitly or explicitly assumes that the patient has either hypochondriatic (i.e., abnormal obsession with the pain) or psychosomatic (i.e., psychological maladjustment to suffering) tendencies. While there is little question that many physicians use these labels to help patients with secondary, emotional pain problems, other physicians use these labels to place blame for their own failures on the patients. This "victim blaming" is apparent when we observe how some physicians, when discussing their problem patients informally, use terms like "crock," "malingerer," or "pain-in-the-ass" to describe those pain patients who are dissatisfied with their physician's effectiveness and, therefore, threaten the doctor's sense of professional esteem.

Whether or not the physician intends to morally discredit the patient, the common reaction among patients is to interpret the term "chronic pain patient" as a negative evaluation of self. They see themselves as somehow being blamed for their misery or as having a weak character for not remaining stoic. To counteract their perceptions of "bad medicine," patients will develop strategies for presenting their cases to physicians in such as way as to keep the focus of the interaction on the pain itself.

Let me cite an example to illustrate this point. Mike is a middle-aged accountant with a long history of cervical (i.e., neck) pain emanating from an automobile accident. At the onset of the problem, Mike was quite open and honest during interactions with his physician:

> I answered all the doctor's questions to the best of my ability. You know, when the pain started, how painful it was, exactly where it hurt, things like that. It seemed natural to cooperate with the guy 'cause he's the doctor, right?

After three unsuccessful surgeries and multiple referrals to a wide range of specialists, Mike was shocked to learn that he was in some way being blamed for his troubles:

> I finally got my doctor to refer me to this neurologist I heard was pretty good. I figured that there might be something going on that the orthopedics were missing. But right off the bat, it looked like we weren't going to make it. . . . He didn't even talk to me much about my neck, just kept harping about how I thought too much about my pain, that I was wasting my time

and was just complaining about something I should just learn to live with!

Bad experiences like this have led Mike to develop a list of strategies to manipulate physicians:

First of all, you never tell a doctor that it hurts only some of the time. If you do, he'll think that your problem is not all that bad. . . . Always tell the doctor that you are using less drugs than you actually do, just to make sure he doesn't think you're just a "popper" looking for a prescription. Act real cheerful in the office. Let them know that you're handling the pain OK. . . . It really seems like they look for any little excuse to send you to a shrink.

Mike's strategies are common throughout the chronic pain subculture. Other strategies to con physicians include complimenting them on their fine reputations in the community (whether or not this is in fact true) and letting them know clearly that one is happy at work and at home in spite of the suffering. It is extremely useful to justify a new consultation by remarking that the pain has just suddenly flared up and appears to be getting worse. In other words, the pain should be presented as representing to some degree a new problem demanding concern, not simply an old problem with which the patient is obsessed.

When strategies for conning the physician break down, open conflict between the two can erupt. I have observed several cases where patients will storm into the office and demand a cure or curse out the physician for being a quack. Threats of malpractice suit can ensue. But the patient ordinarily will attempt to control conflict at this point in the career through interactional strategies Sternbach (1974: 55) refers to as "pain games." As distasteful and ineffective as the relationship may be, the patient may be too dependent upon the power of the physician to prescribe analgesic drugs or legally certify disability to risk breaking off the relationship completely.

VARIATIONS IN THE CHRONIC PAIN CAREER

In addition to the prospect of indefinitely searching for a cure, there are two other (though somewhat unusual) courses of event. Deep depression resulting either from the pain itself or from one's inability to find a cure can lead to suicidal thoughts and attempts. As Wolf (1977: 54) notes:

> The pain person wistfully clings to an inadequate, but heartfelt, conviction that all pain should be short term. Our word choices, then, betray the terrible truth that we simply do not know what to do about persistent pain. As the lady said, cancer would, on the whole, seem preferable. The prospect of there being no end to the experience is so devastating that all but the most determined personality can easily be reduced to a whine and a whimper. And if such a statement seems extravagant, I can only assert that it is not. Yes, some pain persons *do* kill themselves, either in a single act or by degrees, with an overdose or with alcohol.

Wolf's statements do not indicate the fact that the pain must be excruciating before it will lead to suicidal thoughts. Most cases of chronic pain incur light to moderate discomfort. Nevertheless, several physicians (in conversation) have stated that it would be impossible to estimate realistically the number of suicides directly or indirectly resulting from chronic pain because the pain itself is never officially listed as either the cause or motive. Most often, it appears that suicide is accounted for by either depression or some type of physical pathology. Analgesic drug abuse is also an indeterminable factor.

To say that clinical depression is the *cause* of pain-related suicide attempts, though, is to oversimplify the issue, for the person may see positive value in terminating existence. Put simply, the positive value is the total cessation of pain. The irony of pain-related suicide is that it is most likely to occur among people who concur with the medical definition of "chronicity," so total meaninglessness is not an issue. It is attempted by those who give up hope for a cure, but who also feel that they cannot achieve compliance with a central corollary of the medical definition, namely, that the pain-afflicted person is expected to learn to live with the pain. Potential suicides find the awesome reality of the definition of chronicity unmanageable. To illustrate this point, I will cite my own personal experience with a pain-related suicide attempt.

Tom is a 28-year-old university study whom I met when he enrolled in one of my classes. Seven years ago, while he was still in the Navy, Tom developed rheumatoid arthritis and cartilage degeneration in both knees. After repeated surgeries, which have only left him without kneecaps, Tom was given a medical discharge from the Navy along with a partial disability allowance. Tom is in almost constant pain and finds it quite difficult to either stand or sit for any length of time. I interviewed Tom regarding his health problems and the effects the pain was having on his family relations. Tom told me that he would occasionally lapse into mild depression when he would reflect on the effects of the pain on his sex life, especially since he had recently been married. I surmised that Tom was fairly well adjusted to his health problems because he was very interested in doing well in school and was apparently doing quite well in his job as an insurance representative for the Veterans Administration. At the conclusion of our course, I told Tom to call me anytime he felt that something new was developing with his pain problem, but I really didn't expect to hear from him.

Tom called me three months later. He was quite anxious and told me he simply needed someone to talk to. He had attempted suicide the previous evening by swallowing massive amounts of Clineril and Percocet, his regular medications. Just before passing out, he called the police, who immediately rushed him to the hospital. He regained consciousness and proceeded to call me. Tom's depression was the culmination of several factors. First, and foremost, the pain was simply becoming unbearable:

> When you have so much pain for so long, you get tired of it and want to quit coping with it. I almost did it [commit suicide] last week after the V.A. recommended I go for psychiatric evaluation, which really infuriated me. . . . It also made me mad that they can't find out what's the matter with me, so they think it's psychological. But, I said no, I'm feeling that pain.

Second, his wife had just left him. She couldn't put up with his complaining but also, Tom thought, didn't care for the restrictions the pain put on their love making. When I asked Tom how much he thought his family problem contributed to his depression and suicidal attempt, he minimized its effects:

> Sure, my wife was affected, too, by the whole thing. But I didn't, it didn't matter a whole lot. Don't forget that I was married before and got divorced. Mostly because, I think, my first wife wanted me to make more money than I could. . . . I know what you're asking me, but you're wrong. The pain is the number one thing.

A third factor was the Veterans Administration's refusal to promote him to a better and higher-paying job classification because of his excessive absenteeism, which Tom attributed to the fact that he takes so much time off to see doctors.

The positive value of suicide entered Tom's mind about two weeks earlier when he began getting what he considered to be terrible nightmares:

> I had the same dream three or four nights in a row. I saw myself getting out of bed in the middle of the night and grab-

bing this big meat cleaver we keep in the kitchen, and cutting off my legs. I saw my body shrinking as I took off parts to reduce the pain, you know what I mean? But I remember that the pain never went away during the dreams. . . . I don't know how it happened during the dream, but it felt as if I had to cut my whole body away to get rid of all the pain, but that's suicide I guess.

Tom often thought about these nightmares during his waking hours, trying to figure out just how he could kill himself. The meat cleaver seemed too violent, so he threw it out into the trash. He decided on taking an overdose of pills:

Because I got 'em all over the house. I had no idea if they could actually kill me, but I figured they could if I took enough of them.

Until a few days before he attempted suicide, Tom had always believed that *something* could be done for the pain. This belief was shattered when Tom's orthopedic surgeon prescribed a new medication for arthritis. The surgeon was excited about the potential usefulness the drug would have for cases like Tom's. Naturally, Tom was excited too because regular analgesics did very little for him. After a week of using the new drug, Tom realized that it wasn't very effective at all. He perceived the new drug as a last resort and, when it didn't work, he considered suicide as the real last resort.

As we were parting, I asked Tom if he knew someone he could talk to, like a minister or priest, since he didn't want to confront a psychiatrist. He emphatically replied that he didn't believe in God and, besides, he was tired of hearing that his real problem was all in his head. I told him to call me anytime he needed someone to talk to and left it at that. I didn't hear from him for the following three months, so I gave him a call to see how he was doing. His telephone line was disconnected, so I called the Veterans Administration and

talked to Tom's supervisor. He informed me that Tom had
succeeded in killing himself about a month earlier by taking
an overdose of medication.

The analysis of any suicide attempt is always tentative
because precipitating factors and the actor's definition of the
situation are immensely complex, as Douglas (1967) notes,
and Tom's case is no exception. One point is clear, though.
Tom did not have access to any alternative meaning for his
suffering that could supplant the ineffective medical meaning chronic pain.

In addition to suicide, some cases of chronic pain are
resolved by actually being "cured." In the course of doctor
hopping, the person finally may consult a physician who
locates the correct and treatable cause. During my earlier
work with chronic pain (Kotarba, 1975), I encountered Judy,
a 24-year-old college student with severe lower back and leg
pain. Her pain began during her senior year in high school:

> I remember first feeling pain in my legs right after a football
> game my senior year. I was a cheerleader then and I was
> really exhausted. I didn't think too much of it. My daddy said
> I was hurting because I jumped around too much. I supposed
> I believed him [Kotarba, 1975: 155].

As the pain persisted, Judy went from her family physician
to a neurologist and then finally to an orthopedic surgeon.
The orthopedic recommended a laminectomy (i.e., a disc
operation) for what he thought was a ruptured disc. Judy
decided against surgery because her father said she was too
young for such a potentially dangerous course of action:

> The orthopedic doctor said that I needed surgery. Some
> friends of my parents said that back operations leave a lot of
> people crippled. This scared me, so my daddy took me to a
> chiropractor instead. Besides, daddy said that I was too
> young for an operation anyhow [Kotarba, 1975: 156].

When I interviewed Judy, she was currently consulting an acupuncturist from whom, as a point of fact, she was finally obtaining relief. I contacted her six months later to tie up some loose ends in our interview, only to learn that Judy's pain problem had been solved. During a routine physical examination, laboratory tests showed that Judy had a bladder disorder that required surgery. After the surgery, the bladder trouble was not only eliminated, but the back and leg pain disappeared. The surgeon surmises that the infection in the bladder put pressure on certain nerves that radiate into the back area.

Of course, we should consider the possibility of a placebo effect in operation here, by which the surgery distracted Judy from her back and leg pain, making them appear to go away. Nevertheless, Judy was able to avoid unnecessary back surgery and end her pain career successfully. As another example, Bill is a 32-year-old school teacher who found a "cure" after eleven years of back and leg pain and two surgical interventions. Bill thinks that he first hurt his back while playing basketball with several students after school one day. A laminectomy eliminated most of the leg pain, but the back pain continued unabated. After ten years of "hot baths, no lifting, and an occasional aspirin," Bill noticed new pain in the thoracic area. The family physician referred Bill to an orthopedic physician, just to make sure that it wasn't another degenerated disc. The orthopedic physician keenly noticed an unusual spot on the x-rays that he thought may have been arthritic degeneration in the shoulder area, so he referred Bill to a rheumatologist. The rheumatologist did something that Bill had never experienced before: He questioned him concerning the health histories of family members. Bill mentioned that his grandfather and uncle also had back problems. This clue led to a diagnosis of *ankylosing spondylitis,* a hereditary form of arthritis that predominantly strikes males.[20] Laboratory tests verified this diagnosis. The rheu-

matologist immediately placed Bill on a daily regimen of
Indocin, an anti-inflammatory drug. After only one day of
taking the drug, Bill felt complete relief of all pain. The
rheumatologist feels that *spondylitis* was the cause of all the
original pain, and that there was a good chance that Bill
never really had disc trouble, although the symptoms produced by both conditions can be quite similar.

When a pain-afflicted person is fortunate enough to eventually find a cure, any anger previously felt toward medicine
quickly and surprisingly ends. Pain-afflicted people who
spend years cursing the high cost, dishonesty, and ineffectiveness of doctors terminate their diatribes with a simple
sigh of relief. If anything, they remark that their agonizing
experiences have taught them simply to be more careful with
doctors in the future. To heal pain is to heal all related
wounds.

THE FAMILY'S IMPACT ON THE
SEARCH FOR A CURE

The emergence of a chronic pain career cannot be fully
understood without noting the input of the family. Several
writers (e.g., Fordyce, 1976: 115-134; Sternbach, 1974:
56-60) contend that chronic pain can be devastating on
family relations because of the hardships produced by the
selfishness of the pain-afflicted person, loss of income, and
disruption of normal family functions. Furthermore, it is
argued that "tender loving care" offered by the family to the
pain-afflicted person does more harm than good because it
fosters unhealthy dependency in a person who needs to learn
how to cope with the pain problem independently. There
appears to be an implicit assumption among these writers
that chronic pain can only harm the family.

While it is true that some pain-afflicted people do become
unmanageable burdens on their families, this is not univer-
sally the case. Many families do in fact minimize the nega-

tive effects of chronic pain. Indeed, chronic pain can actually have positive benefits for family cohesiveness. The key to understanding this complex phenomenon is whether the family, including the pain-afflicted member, reacts as a *unit* to the pain experience or whether the pain-afflicted person is at odds with other family members over the proper meaning of the pain. In addition, the family can exhibit unity or divisiveness according to the situation at hand.

During the acute stage of the chronic pain experience, the family responds to the suffering just as it would to any type of injury or illness. The individual receives support in seeking health care when it appears that the pain reflects a serious, underlying physical problem. In some cases, the family will suggest health care when the pain persists over time and fails to respond to self-care.

The family's reaction to the pain becomes much more situationally determined, however, when the discomfort is identified as chronic pain. Just as the definition of the pain changes from acute to chronic, the response of the family changes from outright sympathy to a mixture of sympathy and caution. The ongoing search for a cure is usually at the person's initiative. The family will support the search as long as it appears to be reasonable. How reasonable is actually defined depends on family circumstances and the nature of the search. There are three possible criteria for determining whether the family will support a particular venture into the world of health care. First, the intervention should not be too costly. Problems would emerge, say, if a pain-afflicted person from the working class wishes to spend three weeks at an expensive health spa. Well-to-do families tend to exercise less constraint on expensive interventions. Second, the intervention should not be too bizarre according to the family's health care values. If a pain-afflicted Catholic were to decide to attempt fundamental Protestant faith healing, we would expect the family to object. Third, the intervention should not be excessively disruptive. If a parent neglects his or her children in order to meet appointments with various healers, we would expect the other spouse to object.

The search for a cure is not, however, always at the initiative of the pain-afflicted person. The family may initiate a certain intervention if it is perceived as being in the best interests of the family as well as the sufferer. This course of action is most common when secondary pain problems surface, such as analgesic drug abuse and disruptive emotional behavior. In these situations, the pain-afflicted person may not be aware of the problem, but the family will be because it feels it can evaluate the situation more objectively than can the sufferer.

Whether the family reacts to the pain as a unit depends on the effectiveness of communication among its members. In other words, the family will support the search for a cure if it feels that the pain-afflicted member's motives are correct. Correct motives revolve around the desire to eliminate the pain and not around the desire to gain secondary benefits at the expense of the family. For example, the desire to try acupuncture would be sanctioned if the family thought that the pain-afflicted member was seriously interested in it. Above all the family must truly believe that the sufferer really is in serious pain. Since there is usually very little, if any, visible indication that a person is experiencing chronic pain, the effective communication of pain is based on love and trust.

In order for the pain-afflicted person to be assured of family support, he or she must present the impaired self and the symptoms in certain ways. It is most crucial to present the self as being essentially emotionally neutral to the search. By clearly demonstrating that one is not desperate, the pain-afflicted member demonstrates good faith. One of the most effective indications of good faith is the portrayal of the search as being formulated for the good of the family as well as the sufferer. Gary is a 27-year-old mail carrier who slipped on a patch of ice and injured his back several years ago. He has recurrent, severe back pain and engages intermittantly in the search for definitive relief. His wife supports Gary's ventures because she senses Gary's altruistic motives for doing so:

> No, I certainly don't mind Gary going to all these doctors. I know he is in pain. You should see him come home some days, what a mess! He's such a trooper, I can't believe it. I know that he worries all the time about us and what it must be like to live with such a grouch! . . . He's really afraid of what his back might be like in a few years, you know, when the kids will need a father to rough-house with and, you know, show them how to fix cars and things.

A pain-afflicted person who gives the impression that he or she places the pain ahead of family needs risks losing the support of the family. Rachel is a middle-aged housewife who has had lower back pain for the past five years. I talked to her husband one afternoon as he was waiting for her to complete a visit to the family physician:

> Rachel is a strong-headed woman. She usually gets her way, 'bout just about everything. But this acupuncture thing was going too far. I tried to tell her that I thought it was a lot of phooey, sticking a lot of needles in you and all that. . . . Hell, yes, we had a big fight over it! I about had enough. I hollered at her to quit babying herself and think of how we could use that good money for getting the kids back to school, things like that.

If the family reacts as a unit to the pain, all family members can, at times, derive benefit from it. Just as the pain-afflicted person can use the pain as an excuse for neglecting personal responsibilities, the family can use a member's chronic pain to relieve itself of group responsibilities. For example, the father's back may mysteriously "go out" just when the family is expected to attend a party thrown by a cousin who is somewhat less than cherished. This phenomenon is quite similar to the common use of children as excuses for escaping family responsibilities (e.g., "Bobby's been running a fever all day and we couldn't possibly leave him home alone."). In short, the chronic pain experience affects the family identity in ways quite similar to the ways it affects an individual's identity.

Thus we can see that chronic pain doesn't shape family relationships as much as it reflects them. A closely knit family will compensate for the inability of one of its members to perform household chores. A loving wife will excuse her husband's occasional disinterest in sex due to back pain if she has a sense that her marriage is strong. On the other hand, a wife who is having sexual problems with her husband in general may not find the excuse of back pain very convincing.

NOTES

1. Neal (1978: ch. 7) cogently argues that adults underestimate the amount of physical suffering sick children endure. Children feel great pain from terminal diseases such as leukemia, traumatic injuries, burns, and inflicted clinical pain. Bone punctures and marrow aspirations, two procedures directed toward leukemia patients, are especially agonizing. The irony of children's pain results from the rationale behind establishing special dosage levels for children. Low dosages are prescribed in order to minimize the danger of side effects, but lower dosages mean children experience relatively high levels of pain.

2. Nearly all of the health care workers with whom I have worked indicate that back pain is the most common form of chronic pain. The vast majority of pain persons I have encountered have back problems. The overwhelming thrust of the medical, popular, physiological, and rehabilitative literature on chronic pain focuses on back pain. To understand chronic back pain is a necessary step in understanding all forms of intractible pain.

3. Twaddle (1969), among many others, has conclusively demonstrated sociologically what we all take for granted, namely, that pain is the most common symptom leading to the search for medical help.

4. The migraine headache is among the best historically documented forms of chronic pain. The Greeks believed that head pain was caused by the Keres—or evil spirits—which enter a man's stomach and send "humours" to the brain. The Romans believed that a headache was the result of offending a god and being punished for it. Among the famous historical figures who have suffered migraine headaches and have written about them are Friedrich Nietzsche, Charles Darwin, Sigmund Freud, Thomas Jefferson, and Karl Marx (see Mines, 1974: 123-126).

5. The folk concept "slipped disc" so pervades our culture that it is really a commonsense diagnosis, picked up from medical jargon. I have often heard it used in everyday talk as being synonymous with back pain. The concept is fairly recent in origin, emerging during World War II (see Hutchin, 1965: 9-15).

6. As we will see in Chapter 4, most pain patients consult alternative forms of health care only after engaging regular medicine.

7. Physicians routinely make diagnostic, decisions in favor of real illness. Scheff (1966: 105-127) refers to this bias toward illness as a "medical decision-rule." Since the physician believes that he or she works for the good of the patient, he or she would rather impute disease than risk overlooking or missing it.

8. Arthritis patients are usually referred to rheumatologists. Patients with visceral or postoperative pain are referred to internal medicine specialists. Migraine headache patients are referred to neurologists.

9. This is, of course, in addition to the everyday forms of inflicted pain in the hospital setting resulting from intravenous injections, the extraction of blood for laboratory testing, stitching, and so forth.

10. Although myelography is still a popular diagnostic procedure, medical researchers are becoming increasingly skeptical of its validity. As Finneson (1977: 41) notes:

> These studies have a high percentage of abnormalities that are not clinically significant. . . . When pantopaque is introduced into the subarachnoid space for investigation of cervical symptoms or acoustic neurinomas, abnormalities in the lumbar spine have been variously reported in 10% to 25% of patients who have had no low back symptoms. A number of studies have demonstrated that abnormal discograms are unreliable as the patient's age increases. Many spine surgeons place considerable reliance on discograms and myelograms as indicators for surgery. The combination of persisting symptoms and an abnormal discogram and/or myelogram may result in unwarranted back surgery.

11. Traction is routinely applied to back patients with a whole range of symptoms. Yet this therapeutic procedure is apparently of limited value when applied to disc-related pathologies:

> Traction would not have any influence on an inflammatory lesion. How it could help in neck problems is a matter of conjecture. It has the advantage of only applying a distracting force on the joint complex, but it has the disadvantage of being very uncomfortable for the patient (Fisk, 1977: 135).

Nevertheless, many orthopedic physicians prescribe this conservative treatment for those patients who demand intervention but whose symptoms are diagnostically inconclusive.

12. Clinical suicide should probably not be considered a major problem in orthopedic wards, although the evidence clearly shows that it exists. Surprisingly, Wiener (1975) ignores the existence of suicide in her otherwise excellent description of pain management in an orthopedic ward. Her lack of attention to this issue

matches that of the staff she studied, for there is "a tendency for staff to underestimate or disbelieve the degree of pain" (Wiener, 1975: 508).

13. Surgery is rarely recommended for migraine headache patients who are normally kept on high medication regimens or referred to psychiatrists. Arthritis patients are rarely candidates for surgery, although they may incur joint replacements during the latter stages of their careers.

14. Some patients who refuse surgery at this point seek alternative sources of health care, especially chiropractic. Most pain persons who eventually consult alternative healers do so only after running the gamut of medical possibilities.

15. As I have indicated elsewhere (Kotarba, 1977: 265), almost all surgeries of any kind are listed on hospital reports as "successful" if the operating room staff is reasonably confident that the surviving operant leaves surgery without a sponge or two sewn up inside.

16. Physicians can also normalize this residual pain by maintaining that an obtrusive disc can, over time, leave scars on nerve tissue that take a very long time to heal.

17. Traumatic exercise regimens like the Williams program are slowly falling into disfavor among rehabilitative physicians because of the risk of reinjury. Less strenuous regimens like isometrics, isotonics, and stretching exercises are less dangerous and more easily routinized by pain persons (see Kraus, 1970).

18. We cannot ignore the role played by the pharmaceutical industry in the drug abuse issue. The base of the problems lies in medicine's orientation toward treatment of symptoms rather than causes:

> Drug companies spend 750 million dollars per year proselytizing physicians, providing a major part of the post-graduate "education" of physicians. The tranquilizer is a tantalizing temptation to the physician who feels he has exhausted unsuccessfully the alternatives for conventional medical treatment, and the patient goes away, bottle in hand, feeling that the doctor has done something. Meanwhile in the past 25 years, pharmaceutical companies have become the most powerfully effective force in American medicine; their executives are the highest paid group in the country; their profits are in the oil industry league, a good share of the profits being plowed back into the sales effort [Shealy and Shealy, 1976: 22].

19. Williams (1978), among others, argues that the major cause of postsurgical back pain is surgery itself, not any reinjury to the lesion. Adhesions form between the inflicted nerve and surrounding muscle tissue after surgery which continue to pinch the sciatic nerve. During disc surgery, extradural fat (i.e., the tissue that protects the nerve) is lost, thus disrupting the fragile nerve/muscle/bone/cartilege complex.

20. Cousins (1979) provides a personal account of his experience with *ankylosing spondylitis*. He not only relates the tremendous difficulty physicians had in correctly diagnosing his problem, but also describes the great effectiveness of holistic health in reversing the course of his affliction.

4

COMPLEMENTARY HEALTH
CARE MODALITIES

As we have seen, medical intervention is highly influential in shaping the chronic pain career. But it is by no means the only form of health care used by pain-afflicted persons. When medicine is perceived as ineffective in alleviating pain, pain-afflicted people who refuse to believe that their suffering is inherently intractable seek alternative forms of health care, including naturapathy, acupuncture, applied mysticism, and especially, chiropractic. In this chapter we will explore the ways in which pain-afflicted people make use of these services and the reasons why they are perceived as viable alternatives to medicine.

The sociological literature on nonmedical healing is surprisingly sparse.[1] Several writers have examined the occupation of chiropractic (e.g., Cowie and Roebuck, 1975; Rootman and Mills, 1974; White and Skipper, 1971; McCorkle, 1961; Wardwell, 1952), one has looked into the contemporary acupuncture phenomenon (Kotarba, 1975), and another has written on the rationale underlying what she refers to as "quackery" (Cobb, 1958).[2] Skipper (1978: 2-3) has found that general works in medical sociology (i.e., textbooks and edited collections) pay little attention to chiropractic, the most pervasive and influential alternative to medicine in the United States. This situation largely exists because medical sociology suffers from a medical bias (see Gold, 1977). By defining health and health care in a medical framework, most medical sociologists have adopted medical value assumptions. Since organized medicine considers nonmedical healing to be illegitimate and nonscientific, medical sociologists tend to dismiss their importance, if not their very existence.

The few medical sociologists who have analyzed the nonmedical healing arts essentially view them as physicians do: as quackery, but in more scientific-sounding terms like "deviant" (Cowie and Roebuck, 1975) and "marginal" (Wardwell, 1952).[3] It appears that there is something intrinsically wrong or immoral about nonmedical healers and their work. We read that chiropractors, for example, are unscientific, exploitative entrepreneurs who cater to undersocialized, neurotic patients who seek ersatz health care practitioners because they are less expensive but more psychologically comforting than physicians; this is more or less the opinion of organized medicine (see AMA, 1969). Mechanic (1978: 419-421) gives us a grossly distorted portrait of the typical chiropractic patient as a female hypochondriac who requires psychological comforting as well as legitimation of spurious complaints.

The two main sources of data for sociological analyses of nonmedical health care are professional propaganda disseminated by medical and nonmedical health care groups (such as the polemical attacks against nonmedical healing that regularly appear on the editorial page of the *Journal of the American Medical Association,* and surveys of patient utilization of health care services) and direct observation of the delivery and use of nonmedical health care.

Professional propaganda can be misleading. For example, since both types of healers publicly and officially argue that only they can adequately provide *total* patient care, sociologists have assumed that they engage in a winner-take-all battle for patients. We must exercise great caution in interpreting the official propaganda disseminated by health care organizations and lobbying groups. As Altheide and Johnson (1979) have clearly shown, complex organizations manipulate official reports and programmatic statements in order to produce certain public images of their respective groups; this propaganda in no way reflects the reality of how these groups actually accomplish their work. Thus we should be open to the possibility of *accommodation* between the actual members of conflicting health care groups when such a strategy serves them pragmatically.

The validity of sample surveys and official statistics, on the other hand, has been critiqued thoroughly in the sociological literature (e.g., Douglas, 1967). Surveys of health care utilization indicate a distinct overrepresentation of lower- and working-class involvement with nonmedical health care, but they may tell us more about sampling and questioning techniques than about actual health care. It seems quite plausible that middle-class survey respondents may feel too ashamed to admit (even on a questionnaire) that they would actually consult practitioners whom prestigious physicians readily label as *quacks.* I got a sense of this kind of respondent deception during my interviews with pain persons. Lower- and working-class interviewees readily discussed all kinds of medical and nonmedical resources used to treat their pain. Many middle-class interviewees, on the contrary, were quite guarded in formulating their responses to my questions. In a number of cases, middle-class pain persons would not admit that they would even consider seeing, say, a chiropractor, when asked directly. This admission frequently surfaced later in the interview when I made it clear that I would not stigmatize them for admitting that they "cheated" on their physicians. I reassured them by stating that I personally see value in nonmedical health care and have even consulted a chiropractor or two myself.[4]

When we study the actual delivery of nonmedical health care and observe its concrete use by patients, we get an entirely different picture. Since patient utilization of these services is more correctly viewed as situational, they are best conceived of an *complementary health care modalities* (CHCM). Stated differently, most people who consult chiropractors, acupuncturists, and the like do so in search of specific therapeutic goals while maintaining belief in the overall efficacy of medicine. Moreover, social class affiliation simply affects the choice of *which* CHCM to consult, but apparently has little effect on the decision of *whether or not* to consult CHCM at all. Schmitt (1978: 63-65) has called for the analysis of combined use of physicians and chiropractors in light of the existing literature, which falsely posits them as mutually exclusive health care options. Our immediate focus on the chronic pain experience allows us to explore a wide range of medical and nonmedical combinations in use.

The alleged competition between medical and nonmedical healers for the patient's *total* health care simply does not exist. In a nationwide survey, Kuby (1965) found that over 70 percent of the reasons given by patients for going to chiropractors had to do specifically with back pain problems. In my earlier research on acupuncture (Kotarba, 1975: 154-155), I found that approximately 70 percent of acupuncture patients seek help for chronic pain. This percentage is probably higher today, since patient interest in acupuncture for weight loss, hearing problems, and smoking cessation has waned. There is good reason to believe that the people who consult naturapaths, faith healers, and other CHCM represent the same high proportion of pain problems. *It is clear that nonmedical health care in America largely exists because it caters to an eager market composed of medicine's biggest failures: people with chronic pain.* Nonmedical healers may publicly and programmatically state that they offer total health care, but they privately concede occupational dependence on the pain person. One chiropractor explains the situation as follows:

> There is no way any chiropractor can survive without his back patients. We know we can do a lot more for people. . . . The facts of life are that we get the medicos' leftovers, the people who've been butchered up and strung out on drugs. People will come to us for that, but not for any kind of preventive care.

We can safely say, then, that the prevailing sociological analyses of nonmedical health care utilization can be applied, at best, to the small proportion of CHCM patients who use them *exclusively* for all health care needs.

Many chronic pain persons not only consult both medicine and CHCM, but often do so concurrently. In one situation, patients use CHCM exclusively for pain relief while seeing a physician for all other health care needs. They may trust their backs to nonmedical healers, but nothing else:

> You must be kidding! I would never take an illness or *anything serious* to my naturapath. Sure, he can relieve muscle tension in a flash, *but he's still no doctor.* . . . I'm just happy he's good at what he does.

The words "anything serious" are crucial in understanding this evaluation of the naturapath's competence. Chronic pain persons who consult CHCM solely for pain relief view their intervention as the application of a *practical skill.* Back pain is a problem that has to be *managed* rather than *cured* at this late stage of a pain career. As an analogy, going

to a naturapath for a quick rub down is much like taking one's
car to a trusted mechanic for periodic service. The practi-
tioner/client relationship in both cases is service rather than
diagnostically oriented and free of most pretensions. Will, a
38-year-old factory worker with what he refers to as a "bum
back," relates to his chiropractor in such a way:

> I'll go for an adjustment, oh, once every two or three months
> or so. . . . There's really nothing wrong with my back. It just
> goes out every once in awhile. . . . Nah, I don't go for all that
> mumbo jumbo he was laying on me at first. You know, I call
> him "quack" all the time, you know, kidding around. He gets
> a big charge out of it. . . . It's great because I get in and out
> real quick. Snap, snap, here's your ten bucks, and I'm good
> for another couple o' months.

In a second situation, patients use medical and nonmedical health care services concurrently for pain relief. This
situation is largely shaped by the occupational parameters of
medicine and CHCM. A patient, for example, may consult a
physician in order to obtain prescriptions for controlled
medications or for legal validation of continuing disability,
while seeing a chiropractor (who by law cannot prescribe
drugs) for spinal adjustments. During the advanced stages of
a pain career, pain persons can accomplish concurrent con-
sultations because their experience has taught them how to
present managed self-identities. Patients conceal their involvement with CHCM from physicians when it appears
likely that they will be discredited for seeing a quack. It is
much easier to talk to nonmedical practitioners about one's
regular physician because of the mutually acknowledged
underdog status of CHCM:

> After I thought I strained my back painting the bathroom, I
> did go to a chiropractor in La Mesa that my parents had gone
> to, and I got relief. . . . I certainly wasn't getting any relief

from bedrest. . . . I saw my internist a few weeks later. I
wanted so much to tell him that my back pain was gone, but I
decided not to. Let me describe him to you. He's from the old
school and would never approve. . . . Dr. Maritan [the chiro-
practor] asks me everytime I visit about my regular doctor.
He understands my situation and never puts him [the physi-
cian] down. He knows I'll never give up my doctor because of
this thyroid condition.

Some pain patients ask their physicians about the advisability of consulting CHCM when medicine has been ineffective. The stern warnings against CHCM they receive are
sufficient reason to end the discussion and keep any later
involvement with CHCM to themselves:

In April of '74, I had approximately five acupuncture treatments, maybe two weeks apart. . . . I also looked into hypnotism. I, uh, couldn't find anybody I trusted to do it. I got
no support from my doctors about things like that, at all. I
didn't know they would object so vehemently. After that, I
used my own better judgment and kept my mouth shut. . . .
The doctors made me feel ashamed.

If we look beyond the political rhetoric of the medicine/
CHCM controversy, and even beyond specific cases of
mutual condemnation, we learn that many physicians and
nonmedical healers construct accommodating relationships.
In another work, I have shown how physicians specializing
in rehabilitative and physical medicine employ indigenous
acupuncturists (Kotarba, 1975: 165-172). In the present
study, I found several physicians (although certainly the
minority) who consent to CHCM use under two separate
sets of circumstances. First, an open-minded physician may
refer patients to chiropractors or naturapaths when it appears
that the pain is of musculoskeletal origin and could possibly
respond to mild manipulation. Second, a physician may consent to patients' requests for "permission" to see nonmedi-

cal healers either when the physician has exhausted all therapeutic strategies without success or in order to rid him- or herself of malingerers, hypochondriacs, or just plain "pain-in-the-ass" patients (see also Dintenfass, 1973: 47-48).

The essential absurdity of political conflicts between medicine and CHCM emerges clearly when we observe how physicians become chronic pain persons. When the powers of medicine prove to be ineffective for them, paradigmatic barriers collapse and CHCM are redefined as sources of hope for their own pain problems. In all, I have personally encountered seven physicians using various forms of CHCM for stubborn back pain, but who request that my knowledge of their heresy be kept from their watchful peers. Another physician gave up all concern for maintaining professional integrity, for his pain was caused by terminal cancer:

> I have known Phil [the chiropractor] for a long time, six or eight years, I guess. We always got along by, shall we say, extending professional courtesies to each other. [laugh] It seemed like I sent him all my crocks and he sent me all his patients who were really sick. . . . But, you know, it's funny how your world changes. I bet I've seen hundreds of cancer patients in my career. You do what you can for them. . . . I guess you have to look at it scientifically to be able to go home and forget all the misery you've seen that day. . . . Medicine has run out for me. What am I supposed to do, just lay back and die? It's not a hundred lives, it's my life.

A PHENOMENOLOGY OF THE CHIROPRACTIC ENCOUNTER

As we have noted, chiropractic is the largest and most influential of the CHCM. Since its founding in 1895 by Daniel David Palmer, an itinerant grocer and fishmonger, chiropractic has survived the political and scientific onslaught of medicine in the United States (see Wardwell, 1978). Although the sociological literature has been eager to portray the political, scientific, economic, and (alleged) psychological marginality of chiropractors and their patients, it ignores any analysis of the actual chiropractic encounter. The essence of chiropractic lies in the interactive process by which skeptical patients (most of whom are otherwise normal believers in and users of medicine) engage such esoteric healers in order to construct the "spinal adjustment," chiropractic's primary form of therapy. Meaningful intersubjectivity in this situation is really hard work because the spinal adjustment is diametrically opposed to the novice patient's commonsense notions of both the structure of the body and what constitutes proper healing. To understand chiropractic, then, is to see how it becomes a subjectively meaningful health care option for pain persons. Cowie and Roebuck (1975) have made an effort in this direction through the presentation of an ethnographic description of a chiropractic clinic. The authors proposed to study the social definitions held by all actors (i.e., the patient and staff) in and of the chiropractic setting (Cowie and Roebuck, 1975: 9), but actually present data based almost exclusively on the *practitioner's* definitions of the situation. The following is a description of the pain patient's experience of the chiropractic encounter.[5] I have chosen to ignore the experience of those few chronic pain persons who utilize chiropractic for all primary health care and for whom pain is simply one of a number of health problems they present to chiropractors (see McCorkle, 1961). This description is based on the experience of people for whom chiropractic emerges as relevant health care later in their pain careers.

Very few chronic pain persons begin their involvement with chiropractors with any realistic understanding of what chiropractors actually do. Preencounter notions of chiropractors are at best couched in vague terms like "quacks," "back breakers," "back snappers," or "good people to see if you have a bad backache." This imagery has an almost humorous quality to it, for it is difficult to take such low-status pretenders to medicine seriously if they are perceived as irrelevant to one's own pain problems. But treating the idea of chiropractic with levity is also a reflection of the more general, cultural view of the "bad back" phenomenon as the object of jokes, cartoons, and satire (e.g., Snoopy, in contemplating pain from the roof of his doghouse: "I always thought you got a headache because your ears were too tight!").

Chiropractic becomes consciously relevant to an individual when certain conditions are met. The pain-afflicted person must be in search of alternatives to existing pain care strategies that are not working. The person must also feel confident that the pain is not caused by disease, internal injury, or other organic pathologies best left to a physician. Since chiropractic is usually suggested by a friend or relative, the individual responds with three types of questions: (1) "What will he do to me?" (2) "Will the treatment itself be painful?" and (3) "Can the treatment make my problem worse?" Answers given to the first question are rarely satisfactory because it is quite difficult to explain in common-sense terms just what an adjustment really is. Typical answers include: "He'll snap your back just like you crack your knuckles." "He'll bend you around until your back is straight and in place." These responses make little sense to the individual because the experience of embodiment indicates that pain may be caused by something broken in the back, but not by something supposedly out of place in an area of the body experienced as a solid, if flexible, structure.

Although the definitional framing of the adjustment may leave the individual skeptical of the whole matter, negative responses to the next two questions are sufficient reason for deciding to see a chiropractor. As long as the sufferer is assured that chiropractic won't hurt and won't make the problem worse, an evaluation voiced as: "What do I have to lose?" (implied answer: "nothing") emerges. But enough skepticism of chiropractic in general remains to preclude simply picking a practitioner randomly out of the telephone directory. Most individuals consult chiropractors whom significant others have found, through personal experience, to be competent.[6] This strategy is simply a way of minimizing the risk of the unknown.

Preparation for the chiropractic encounter is shaped largely by one's previous experience with physicians. A bath, clean clothes, clean underwear, and a coherent account of the history of the problem are perceived as prerequisites for the presentation of competency.

Prior expectations of chiropractors, are immediately shaken on entry into the office, however. Chiropractic offices tend to be relatively old, plain, and minus the usual trappings found in a physician's office. The chiropractor's competence is questioned when framed by the unprofessional atmosphere of the setting, for as one pain person noted: "I went inside and said what kind of doctor *is* this?" Chiropractic literature is available in the waiting area and eagerly surveyed in hope of finding out more about what is to come. But the literature is of little use to the novice patient because, like the explanations of chiropractic received from confidants, it is also quite vague. For example, a brochure titled "Arm and Shoulder Pain" discusses a number of different causes for pain such as bursitis and radiculitis. In a total of eight pages, however, the only statements indicating what the chiropractor can do for these causes are the following:

> Fortunately, the doctor of chiropractic is emminently qualified to correct arm and shoulder problems, better qualified than any other kind of doctor.
>
> The chiropractor's education and experience have been spine, nerves, muscles and joints of the human body.
>
> Today's doctor of chiropractic first seeks to give you immediate relief, but his education and experience cause him to

always seek the *underlying cause* of your problem and correct it.[7]

In other words, an aura of mystery pervades the setting.

The patient's first impression on entering the inner office and meeting the chiropractor is that the chiropractor does not look like a doctor. Most chiropractors dress fairly casually—the lack of the physician's white smock is noticeable. (The patient will later learn that the chiropractor's casual dress is necessary in light of the difficult, physically strenuous work incurred by the adjustment.) The patient is surprised to learn that the chiropractor does not *talk* like a physician either. Instead of encountering the abrupt and impersonal manner of physicians, the patient actually feels ill at ease when the chiropractor talks leisurely about the entire history of the problem. This discomfort is compounded by the fact that the chiropractor spends considerable time (perhaps twenty to thirty minutes) talking about the faults of medicine (of which the individual is already quite aware) and the *theory* of chiropractic, ignoring totally any discussion of actual chiropractic procedures and treatments. Chiropractors routinely take x-rays of the patient's back on machinery that may appear to be old and archaic, unlike the technologically elaborate and aesthetically pleasing apparatus found in a hospital radiology unit. Whether or not x-rays are taken, the chiropractor inevitably finds something out of place in the spine. Diagnoses (or "analyses," as chiropractors prefer to call them[8]), such as "a subluxation of the vertebra," make little sense to the patient. The chiropractor may demonstrate the diagnosis on a plastic model of the spinal column, indicating how a malaligned vertebra can pinch a nerve, resulting in pain. This demonstration is much more meaningful to the patient than the strictly verbal explanations, which sound like "a bunch of mumbo jumbo," as they are often described. The demonstration actually shows that the spinal column is segmented, a reality not discernible simply through embodied experience.

The patient's anxiety increases when led into the treatment area. Unlike a physician's treatment area, which is filled with cabinets full of medications, counters arranged with syringes and tongue depressors, and calendars imprinted with the logos of pharmaceutical companies, the chiropractor's work space contains little more than a long, adjustable treatment table. The pain person is surprised to learn that he or she is not required to disrobe for the adjustment. It does not seem possible that the chiropractor can do anything without direct visual and tactile contact with one's body.

The patient is instructed to lie flat on the table stomach down. As the chiropractor maintains continuous talk (about nearly anything), he or she massages the back, either manually or with the aid of an electric vibrator, for three to four minutes. The massage in itself is pleasurable if not pain relieving. The practitioner then consels the patient to relax because, as is said, "This won't hurt a bit, but the adjustment won't take if you are tense." This directive, needless to say, has an opposite meaning for the patient whose previous experience with health care workers has shown that it *always* hurts when the doctor or nurse says it won't (see also Fagerhaugh and Strauss, 1977: 97-98).

The chiropractor then runs his or her fingers up and down the spine in order to locate the proper point for the adjustment. There are several different types of adjustment, depending on location on the spinal column. If the adjustment is made in the thoracic area (i.e., between the shoulders), the chiropractor lays one palm on the vertebra is question and, with the help of the other hand, thrusts inward quite sharply. If the adjustment is made in the cervical area (i.e., the neck), the chiropractor will simply clasp the head on either side with both hands and sharply twist the head, usually in both lateral directions. Adjustments made in the lumbar area (i.e., low back) are somewhat more intricate, requiring movement of the legs as well as the back.

The patient is thankful that the actual adjustment takes so little time, for it can be a somewhat terrifying experience. The subjective sensation of an adjustment is really less of an audible "pop," as Cowie and Roebuck (1975: 89) have described it, than a crunching and tearing feeling. The pain patient momentarily thinks that the chiropractor might have broken something, but is relieved when the chiropractor states that the adjustment was successful. Still, the patient treats the adjusted area quite gingerly for awhile until he or she feels confident that nothing was really damaged.

After several minutes of postadjustment rest, the patient and practitioner are again sitting in the office together. The patient gladly pays the 10- or 15-dollar fee because it is ridiculously inexpensive compared to the 50- to 75-dollar fee required to see a medical specialist for a few minutes of his or her precious time. The chiropractor will, at this point, suggest that the patient may need a series of adjustments in order to correct a stubborn condition, and that it is cheaper to enroll in a family plan that guarantees complete preventive and corrective care for the patient and his or her "loved ones." All patients openly respond that "they will keep that in mind," but most privately realize that this is the chiropractor's "sell job" that everyone warned them about. The fact is that most pain persons won't return for follow-up treatments unless the first or possibly second adjustment actually relieves the pain.

After the first encounter with chiropractic, the pain-afflicted person is able to place the whole experience into perspective. The patient realizes that he or she really paid for a short and simple service that does not appear to require much training. All the talk surrounding the adjustment seems pretty useless to most patients who realize that the chiropractor must "dress up" his or her work in order to present an identity of professional competence and to earn one's fees. Veteran chiropractic patients can, by demonstrating knowledge and acceptance of the phenomenon, manipulate successive encounters in order to eliminate the useless talk and quickly receive an adjustment.

The issue of whether or not chiropractors can actually relieve pain by realigning the spinal column is not within the scope of this work. Only focused medical research can answer this question. Most pain-afflicted people I've talked with feel that their encounters with chiropractic have been of either "some" or "little" help. But if we control for the therapeutic effectiveness of chiropractic, we are still faced with certain residual or secondary benefits of the chiropractic encounter. Pain-afflicted people, over time, acquire the habit of pampering the painful area. The natural reaction is to minimize any exertion placed upon the lesion. For the person with back problems, this conservative reaction is counterproductive because it often leads to physical inactivity, which further weakens the damaged area and increases the risk of reinjury and musculoskeletal degeneration (Fordyce, 1976: 57-60). The traumatic essence of the spinal adjustment indicates to many individuals that their backs can indeed take high levels of exertion without incurring further damage. In this regard, the chiropractic encounter can be a catalyst for reengagement with normal activity and even the exercise regimen so important to the rehabilitation of damaged tissue.

But even more telling is the long-term effect of the chiropractic encounter on the career of the pain-afflicted person. For many sufferers, the chiropractic encounter marks the first true "break" with the medical definition and control of the pain. By summoning the courage to try a health care recourse as esoteric as chiropractic, the patients prove to themselves and others that they can regain control over the fate of their pain and their bodies. They now have a criterion with which to evaluate their previous experience with medicine; for better or for worse, they can accept the possibility that effective pain relief just might be found by locating the appropriate *type* of healer and not by locating the appropriate *medical* healer, as has been their strategy in the past.[9]

APPLIED MYSTICISM

In addition to chiropractic, osteopathy, and other long-established health care modalities that have experienced a renaissance due to the emergence of the chronic pain phenomenon,[10] a number of new forms of pain care have been established to meet the demands of the market. Since these forms of CHCM are based on holistic notions of self-activated, cognitive control of embodied experience, I refer to them as *applied mysticism*. Religion (sometimes in the form of faith healing), meditation, biofeedback, self-actualization, acupuncture, and hypnosis all fall under this conceptualization.

Simply speaking, applied mysticism is *the promotion of transcendental or metaphysical belief systems for pain control through the accomplishment of a higher state of consciousness.* In general, these belief systems existed long before their proponents became aware of their applicability to pain management. As with all religions and metaphysical movements, their traditional twofold function has been the exploration and explanation of the sacred and the supernatural (see Johnstone, 1975: 12-24). The ideas and practices of these belief systems have in recent years been applied to pain management as a *practical* problem for two interrelated reasons. First, the normalization of human suffering has always been within the province of transcendental belief systems. In this regard, chronic pain is seen as simply another form of physical suffering for which these belief systems can offer comfort and meaning. Second, a profit motive lies at the center of many of their claims to expertise in pain management. Proponents of applied mysticism benefit both by attracting new "converts" to their laity through specific success in pain management and by charging fees for their ser-vices. In the more secular forms of applied mysticism such as acupuncture, one need not become a true believer in order to obtain pain services, but need only pay the required fees.

From the chronic pain person's perspective, applied mysticism may not only alleviate pain but may provide certain *meaning* for pain that helps the person cope with physical suffering. When the efforts of medicine fail, physicians rarely tell their patients how to live with pain (see Mines, 1974: 2). The pain person, then, is left alone in a state of absurdity. The pain's previous meaning—a transitory ailment that at some point would be healed or cured—evaporates. At this point in the pain career, the pain is commonly perceived by the person as a treacherous onus fused to the core of one's embodied existence. The pain person may find it quite difficult, if not impossible, to conceive of the pain rationally and objectively. It is now less referred to as *the* pain than as *my* pain. A sense of isolation accompanies the awareness that the pain not only makes no sense to the individual but is also in phenomenological terms a nonreality to those trusted to make sense of such matters.

Applied mysticism's promise of hope evolves from its general assumption that there are two kinds of existence: *embodied* and *spiritual* (Yinger, 1971: 146-147). Embodied existence is imperfect because it is constrained by the limits of the flesh, Original Sin, and/or the dictates of a material world, which provide little or no understanding of the "true" purpose of life. Spiritual existence, if developed consciously and methodically, escapes the material world by aligning the individual with a unity or a vision of truth that transcends corporality.[11] Embodied pain may still exist, but is no longer in need of mundane (i.e., scientific or medical) sense making. Pain is left behind, along with other worldly concerns, on the road to spiritual fulfillment. Of course, this intriguing proposition is not new, for men have always sought refuge from the absurdity of an imperfect world. But the contemporary use of applied mysticism for pain control is distinctly marked by a fusion of ancient metaphysical ideas with the contingencies of modern social life, technology, and the media. I will describe briefly several forms of applied mysticism and their application to chronic pain management.

Religion is the most common form of applied mysticism. Organized religion has through the centuries provided a spiritual escape from the political, economic, and physical suffering of everyday life. Christianity is most notable in attributing a *positive* sense to physical pain. Whereas the Old Testament repeatedly speaks of suffering as a form of punishment, the New Testament ascribes a religious significance to suffering within the framework of God's plan of salvation for mankind:

> The central point is the Passion of Our Lord. The idea of vicarious suffering adumbrated in the Book of Isaiah finds its practical fulfillment in the Passion and Death of the Lord and Savior Jesus Christ. In consequence, all suffering now becomes a suffering with Christ and takes on the character of redemption [Sauerbruch and Wenke, 1963: 129].

For the Christian believer, pain and physical suffering are God's way of testing, strengthening, and purifying His children. The good Christian is expected to endure pain patiently and offer it in sacrifice for one's sins. But Christianity also teaches that spiritual unity with God can actually reduce the suffering of pain by redirecting one's attention to a higher good, as Thomas Aquinas explains in his discussion of martyrdom: "The holy pleasure of contemplating divine things diminishes physical pain; and the martyrs suffered their pains more patiently because they were completely suffused with the love of God" (1964: 115). This does not mean to say that the Christian should refuse pain alleviation when available; man is instructed to obey the life-preserving laws of science as well as the spiritual laws of God. Nevertheless, pain is viewed as the normal consequence of the fall from grace (i.e., Original Sin) and should be accepted as normal.

Christian views on pain and suffering are promulgated through personal channels such as the pulpit as well as the public media channels used to spread the gospel (see also Atheide and Johnson, 1977: 344-345). From an informal survey of Christian literature and media programming, it appears that illness and pain are among the most common personal problems directed to Christian leaders. In Billy Graham's syndicated newspaper column, he often answers questions pertaining to illness and pain in ways obviously designed to encourage readers to view their suffering as a blessing from God:

Q. I have been a Christian all my life, but now I am in constant pain because of an illness. It seems like it is so hard to even think about God when my life is filled with pain. Is this normal?

A. Pain can seem to block out everything else, including our thoughts about God. However, that does not mean we should resign ourselves to it. Throughout the ages there have been countless saints of God who have found that pain and sickness became a blessing instead of a barrier. They found it could actually help get life into its true perspective.

Think of the apostle Paul. He seldom speaks about his physical ills—which should, incidently, tell us we should not become too absorbed in our own problems and turn our eyes therefore away from Christ. And yet he apparently had some type of painful illness which plagued him and made his ministry more difficult.

He tells us that he begged the Lord to take it away three times, but each time the Lord said "no" to his prayer. Through that experience he came to see in a new way how important it was to rely completely on Christ instead of his own strength. "Therefore, I have cheerfully made up my mind to be proud of my weaknesses, because they mean a deeper experience of the power of Christ . . . my very weakness makes me strong in him" [2 Corinthians 12: 9-10, Phillips translation].

It may seem hard to thank God for your pain. But ask God
to teach you whatever He wants of you during your time.[12]

Pain-afflicted people who adhere strongly to the Christian
normalization of pain are, simply speaking, Christian in
their overall religious attitudes. They consult their ministers
and priests for help in coping with pain just as they would for
other "spiritual" (read: psychological or interpersonal)
problems. Betty is a middle-aged elementary school teacher
who has suffered from rheumatoid arthritis for 27 years. She
has received the moral strength to endure her pain from her
religion and her family minister:

> I've been a Baptist all my life, raised that way. . . . I don't let
> myself get too worried about my arthritis because Jesus suf-
> fered and died for me, so why shouldn't I suffer for Him? But,
> you know, I know I couldn't go it alone without Reverend
> Higgins. He's been such a sweetheart all these years. When
> I'm ready to give up, he has a way of cheering me up. . . .
> Reverend Higgins prays with me and reminds me of the
> rewards I'll get in heaven.

Betty is like most other Christian sufferers, however, in that
she regularly consults medicine for pain relief while obtaining emotional and spiritual support from her religion.

A certain minority of Christian sufferers actually seek
healing through their religion. They are members of the
Pentacostal Church, Christian Science, and other sects that
officially reject medicine and rely solely on prayer and divine
intervention for health care. The studies by Allen and Wallis
(1976: 50-51), Nudelman (1976: 123-24), and others indicate, however, that members of these groups do consult
medicine when it appears that illness or pain is serious. My
own contact with pain-afflicted people who truly believe in
faith healing is limited, but I have found that it is used only by
persons with either mildly or extremely problematic pain.
Faith healing fits mildly problematic pain such as arthritis

among the elderly because a person can realistically hope for either direct healing or, more likely, the pleasure of receiving total relief from dying a Christian death:

> I pray to God everyday to take away my pain. . . . My arthritis flares up really bad when it gets damp outside. . . . No, I don't think God has forsaken me. Look, He just chooses some people to suffer on earth. I'll just be thankful if He gives me the strength to die a Christian, too.

At the other extreme, individuals who are desperate for help may engage in what I call the *Fatima phenomenon.* In this situation, the pain person no longer seeks any type of normal healing, but instead pursues a miraculous cure. These unusual cases are best documented by perusal of the display of charismatic healing on televised Christian ministries (e.g., *Oral Roberts, Jimmy Swaggert,* and *The PTL Club*).

Meditation, biofeedback, and *autogenic training* are all variations of the same process. In short, they direct the individual toward conscious control of body processes and the voluntary alleviation of pain. Compared to religion, which directs a person's consciousness toward an external deity, meditation and its derivatives direct a person's consciousness inwardly, to the self of God (see Weil, 1972: 35-36). The main difference among these regimens is that meditation is religious in tone while the others are distinctly secular.

Meditation

Although Western religious history is rich with examples of the use of meditative techniques to achieve ascetic states (e.g., St. Paul and Thomas Merton),[13] contemporary interest in this experience is largely derived from Eastern teachings (Bellah, 1976: 341). The counterculture movement of the 1960s did much to introduce Eastern thinking into the United States, along with its unique perspective on pain and suffering. There are many types of meditation available (e.g., Transcendental Meditation and Zen Buddhism); we shall focus on Siddha Yoga as a relatively simple yet popular form of self-actualization.

Siddha Yoga is the work of Swami Muktananda Paramahansa (Baba), an Indian guru who first visited the West in 1970. His form of meditation is easily learned because it evolves from one universal mantra, as opposed to other forms of meditation that require specific mantras for each meditant. Meditation is a means for reaching unity with one's self by experiencing the "true" self, which is a microcosm of the universe. The true self is a being untouched by the material or social order:

> To find the place of our true strength we have to be able to transcend everything that our culture and our upbringing have made us think is us. In meditation we go deep beneath all the accidental circumstances of our life, behind our personalities, our life-dramas and hopes and fears, down to that which is before all: a simple sense of being. Our personality has its foundation here, and it is from here that it must draw its strength. It is a strong place, unmoved by concern for what others think or say, oblivious to questions of status of sex or disease or wealth or power. The same formless being dwells within every person and is each person's root [Muktananda, 1976: 30].

The chant used to transcend normal consciousness and to enter Tandra (i.e., the state of high consciousness in which one sees invisible things and comprehends incomprehensible mysteries) reads, "OM Namah Sivaya," or in English, "Hail to the Inner Self." Tandra is a state of perfect happiness, where disease and pain cease to exist:

> The state of tandra is always blissful. Just as you experience the waking state in the gross body, you experience the tandra state in the subtle heart centre. You fall into a sort of wakeful sleep. Tandra is very beneficial. It gives strength to the body,

senses and mind. It enables you to overcome many diseases: certain ailments automatically disappear and inner happiness increases. . . . Pain can be felt only in a certain state. It cannot reach all the states. Pain can never touch your inner perfect being [Muktananda, 1974: 3-4, 55].

It is ironic that the person in pain may encounter esoteric meditation through public educational services. A high proportion of students enrolled in classes in meditation offered through YMCAs and university extension/adult education systems are there specifically to obtain meaning for suffering. As an illustration, the extension service of Wilson University[14] offered a weekend seminar titled: "Meditation: A Journey Into Now." For 43 dollars, students were taught the art of Siddha meditation by a psychotherapist (accredited by a Masters of Social Work degree) who is also director of a private center for the study of the self. The 34 students present were about equally divided between adult men and women. Of the 34 students, 18 enrolled primarily to learn a new technique for managing their chronic pain.[15] As a group, these individuals held very little interest in the religious aspects of Siddha meditation. They were simply intrigued by the class announcement that read: "Siddha meditation is a simple way to relieve the aches and pains that impinge upon our hectic lives." These veteran sufferers made the cognitive link between this path to relaxation and their prior understanding, obtained through discussions with others and through reading the popular literature on pain management, that pain can be alleviated through relaxation techniques. Jill is a 35-year-old nurse administrator who hurt her back lifting a patient several years ago:

Being a nurse, I've seen how medicine can really make a back problem worse. I've been lucky to avoid surgery, even though it's been suggested a number of times. . . . I've tried TM, autogenics, hypnosis, all the fads. I need to relax when I get home. . . . After a day at the hospital, I'm pretty well shot.

Several students indicated that they became interested in learning meditation through the university extension because other sources of this skill were very expensive and extremely cultish:

> When I talked to the guy at TM, I almost died. I couldn't believe what they were charging. . . . My gut feeling is that all these meditations are pretty much the same, and you know how cheap extension classes are . . . and, I don't have to put up with a bunch of hippies who want to see God. . . . If you'll look around, you'll see a lot of people here just like me.

During the seminar, the pain students followed directions and participated just like the other students. The differences in purpose surfaced during the question-and-answer periods that dotted the two-day seminar. Whereas the nonpain students were primarily concerned with the religious and philosophical aspects of Siddha Yoga, the pain students asked questions about the medical and physiological dimensions of meditation. For example, they would ask about the relationship of Siddha meditation and high blood pressure, a factor in migraine headaches. As a group, the pain students were somewhat disappointed when the instructor attempted to avoid this sort of mundane discussion and preferred to talk about levels of consciousness and the teachings of the gurus. Finally, the pragmatic pain students quickly caught on to the instructor's "business hustle." At the end of the seminar, he suggested that all participants enroll in regular meditation classes offered at his study center. The skepticism that develops over years of searching for help and meaning left the pain students weary of rip-offs:

> It's the same old thing. When they hear that you're here because of your back trouble, they know you're probably desperate. Just like my old chiropractor who wanted me there three times a week. . . . You wouldn't mind so much if they were really curing you, no, as a matter of fact, you'd do anything they say if they were curing you. But, c'mon, this is not Mayo's clinic.

In spite of the shortcomings of the meditation seminar, the pain students almost all felt that it was worth the time and money. They not only got a chance to try something new in the long search for help, but also enjoyed involvement with this aspect of the chronic pain subculture. During lunch and coffee breaks, the pain students formed small groups that allowed them to compare notes. I drifted in and out of these informal sessions and heard much discussion regarding the effectiveness of various types of relaxation therapy, the word on new specialists in town, pain biographies, and other topics of interest for pain students.

Biofeedback and Autogenic Training

Biofeedback and autogenic training are two major forms of *secularized* meditation. While inspired somewhat by the therapeutic success of religious meditation, they are structured and explained by Western scientific concepts. Biofeedback training

> is the procedure that allows us to tune into our bodily functions and, eventually, to control them. . . . In a typical biofeedback training session a subject is given this feedback by hooking up with equipment that can amplify one or another of his body signals and translate them into readily observable signals: a flashing light, the movement of a needle, a steady tone, the squiggle of a pen. Once a person can "see" his heartbeats or "hear" his brain waves, he has the information he needs to begin controlling them [Karlins and Andrews, 1972: 24-25].

Subjects learns to control their body processes in ways similar to meditation. Conscious relaxation of specific body parts (e.g., tense back muscles) or body processes (e.g., blood pressure) can be monitored by electroencephalographic or electromyographic apparatus. Unlike meditation, though, biofeedback requires little self-discipline and no appreciation for the esoteric.

Autogenic training, or self-hypnosis, is one very popular way of inducing inner calm and relaxation in conjunction with biofeedback monitoring (Pinkerton et al., 1982: 342-346). It was developed in 1910 by a German named Johannes Schultz and is widely practiced in Europe. Subjects are taught to relax voluntarily specific body parts in succession. For example, one may begin by silently repeating: "my toes are heavy and warm" then "my knees are heavy and warm" and so forth until every major body part, especially the painful areas, is consciously reflected on. Whereas it is asserted that meditation leads to contact with the eternal or the universal, biofeedback and autogenic training simply assert that one can shift patterns of brain activity. By concentration, one can move from beta wave patterns, which mark normal waking activity, to alpha waves, which characterize the passive, relaxed, and tranquil state of mind and body.

Melzack and Chapman (1973: 1) have noted biofeedback's implications for pain control:

> This method appears to be effective for self-regulation of pain. Subjects are trained to increase the amount of alpha brain rhythm by providing a feedback signal (such as a tone) whenever alpha rhythms appear in their electroencephalogram. A high degree of alpha rhythm is associated with meditational states. The evidence so far is suggestive. Gannon and Sternbach reported that a subject who received alpha training was able to delay onset of migraine headaches by self-induction of the alpha state, but was unable to modify the pain after it was under way.

Melzack and Chapman indicate four possible ways biofeedback may relieve pain. First, the individual's attention to pain may be distracted by concentration on the signal. Second, the technology may induce the power of suggestion or self-hypnosis. Third, the relaxation that accompanies the alpha state helps diminish pain by decreasing anxiety and the perception of pain. Fourth, the development of a sense of control over the pain promotes assurance and diminishes anxiety, and with it, pain.

Unlike meditation, these secular forms of self-actualization are encountered through more normal channels of health care. They are important elements in the pain control center program. I will discuss the patient's experience of these modalities in the following section on pain control centers.

Acupuncture

Acupuncture is a hybrid form of applied mysticism. It is an ancient form of oriental healing that involves the insertion of long, slender needles into various parts of the body.[16] Acupuncture is based on the Eastern philosophy of mind/body unity. Accordingly, disease is thought to be a manifestation of imbalance between Yin (male) and Yang (female) energy flows. The insertion of needles removes "blocks" in the energy flow that lead to imbalance.[16] The larger purpose of oriental acupuncture is to restore harmony not only between body and mind, but also among man and heaven and earth (see Mann, 1973).

Unlike other forms of applied mysticism, however, acupuncture requires the active intervention of a practitioner. In another work (Kotarba, 1975), I have shown how acupuncture is being coopted by American health care workers and adopted into the practices of physicians, chiropractors, osteopaths, and the like. The health care workers either learn the art themselves (usually without consenting to its underlying philosophical connotations) or hire indigenous acupuncturists to provide this service. Like biofeedback and autogenic training, acupuncture is practiced in many pain centers.

THE CHRONIC PAIN CENTER

The chronic pain center is a relatively new concept in pain care. Dr. John J. Bonica, an anesthesiologist, started the first pain center in Seattle at the University of Washington Hospital in 1961. Bonica's clinic grew out of the normal procedure by which he would regularly consult neurosurgeons, orthopedic physicians, psychiatrists, nurses, and medical social workers in attempts to solve complicated chronic pain problems:

> And soon it came about that I was getting these people together in conferences, informal conferences, and found that this interaction and personal exchange was effective when it cleared many things up for us. So I began to talk about this pain clinic concept [quoted in Mines, 1974: 54].

Bonica's concept was slow to catch on in the world of pain care. It wasn't until the early 1970s, when chronic pain emerged as a medical phenomenon, that the idea spread. Today, there are more than 800 pain centers in the United States and it appears that most major hospitals soon will have some sort of pain care unit.[17]

Most pain centers are auxiliary units of existing health care facilities. Likewise, most centers are interdisciplinary in staffing and philosophy, and a few are administered by nonmedical personnel such as nurses and clinical psychologists. They are usually organized in terms of outpatient care. And they are expensive. A typical five-day course may cost anywhere from 1000 to 5000 dollars.

There is variation among pain centers in terms of services offered. A few centers concentrate on specific treatments such as nerve blocks and transcutaneous electrical stimulation (TES), or specific types of pain problems such as migraine headaches or back disorders. Others, which are truly interdisciplinary and on which we will focus, treat both the physiological and psychological effects of chronic pain in somewhat holistic fashion. There is an underlying philosophy to the pain center concept. They offer help in coping with pain to the person who has run the gamut of medical interventions, who has probably acquired an unhealthy analgesic drug habit, and whose pain disrupts normal activities and relationships. Pain center administrators claim that their programs offer the best hope for managing intractable pain (e.g., Freese, 1974: 31). Pain center patients approach the centers with (occasionally unrealistically) high expectations of success. The following is an analysis of the actual *experience* of being a chronic pain center patient.[18] It is a composite portrait, drawing on patient experiences in a range of different kinds of pain centers. My primary emphasis, however, is on those centers that organize their work around behavior modification techniques. This apparently is the dominant form of organization and philosophy in the field.

Patients can learn of the pain center option from two sources. First, their physicians may refer them to local pain centers, either directly or through the insistence of disability insurance carriers seeking to absolve themselves from problem clients. Second, they may hear of this option through involvement with the chronic pain subculture. Informal conversations with other sufferers and media coverage are common sources for this information. In general, patients have high expectations for their encounters with the pain center, in spite of warnings from pain center personnel to the contrary. The modal expectation is *total* pain relief:

> I thought that my expectations of help had become very realistic. I gave up the notion of finding that cure and figured that any help was worth any amount of effort. But in the back of my mind, I still felt that, hey, maybe this pain center thing was really it. Maybe these doctors had the answer.

Pain center administrators establish rules for patient eligibility. In general, the pain must be of long duration (usually six months or longer[19]) and there must not be any apparent organic pathology causing the pain that could be remedied by surgical intervention. Patients must be committed to participation and cooperation with the program. And the patient must demonstrate the ability to pay. In addition, several pain centers require formal referral from a physician.

These eligibility rules appear more rigid than their actual implementation. The prospective patient soon learns that the most crucial requisite for admission is the ability to pay. This is not to say that the pain centers operate solely on a profit basis. But they do operate on fairly marginal budgets. They draw much of their staff on a part-time basis from other hospital departments, an exceptionally costly process. In addition, interdisciplinary care requires many different, highly specialized, and highly paid workers. The net result is that *the greatest proportion of pain center patients are referred and funded by disability compensation carriers.*[20] Administrators may deny admission to people currently engaged in litigation, though, because of the high energy, time, and emotional costs of court involvement.

The duration of pain and the physician's referral are, practically speaking, secondary and occasionally irrelevant criteria. By the time a pain-afflicted person is in the desperate position of even considering an expensive alternative like the pain center, he or she can easily obtain referral from a frustrated physician.

At the beginning of the program, patients undergo a series of evaluations and screenings. The program director (or the patient's personal program manager in some centers) elicits a detailed medical history. A physician examines the patient to make sure that no underlying yet remediable pathology is present. A medical social worker elicits a family history, searching for examples of how the pain may be disrupting family responsibilities. An occupational therapist may discuss the patient's work history, work environment, and potentially reusable work skills if the patient is currently unemployed.

The clinical psychologist plays a central role in those centers that stress behavioral or operant conditioning interventions. As noted in Chapter 2, clinical psychologists are trained to find personality disorders resulting from pain, even when the subject may be considered (and self-defined as) "normal." Objective personality inventories are administered to verify these clinical expectations. The most popular of these tests is the Minnesota Multiphasic Personality Inventory (MMPI). While it is true that the internal validity of the MMPI is the subject of heated debate (see Butcher, 1969), the clinical validity of the test is distorted by the patients' perception of the test. For example, completion of the test is commonly haphazard:

> I was in the psychologist's office my first day to take some tests. That was the day I took the MMPI. And I'm sitting with a fellow who was entering the program with me. . . . He kept on laughing about all the questions. And I said [to myself]: "Oh, this nurd, he's never taken a test like this before." . . . And he said: "This is ridiculous. . . . What do they want to know this for? . . . Why would this pertain in any way with anything wrong with my back?"

This kind of skepticism is common among many pain center patients who, in their naive ways, understand that the staff is questioning their selves (i.e., character and integrity) and not simply focusing on the pain per se. Skeptical patients put less than total effort and concentration in completing what they see as silly tests.

Other patients, usually with some testing experience and a little knowledge of pop psychology, attempt to construct their responses in such a way as to "psych out" the tester and prove that there is nothing wrong with them psychologically:

> I tried to show them that there was nothing wrong with me, that I'm all right. . . . that I don't think there's a strange person coming after me and I don't think about my pain in my dreams. . . . I thought they were trying to find out how much of my pain was psychological. Well, I *know* my pain is not

psychological. . . . I know a lot of us tried to out-psych the
test. We may be desperate, but we're no dummies.

Needless to say, the testers are largely unaware of the patients' manipulation of the tests. They assume that all patients are conscientious and objective. There are, in fact,
good patients who are conscientious during the test, just as
they are totally cooperative during the remainder of their
pain center experience. Even the good patients, however,
may be shocked to learn that, although their test results indicate no evidence of personality disorder, the psychologist
may refuse to believe it:

> The psychologist said that everything was *too* good, that
> everything looked *too* good on my test. And that my husband
> couldn't be *that* good to me. And my relationships couldn't
> be that good. . . . He kept asking: "What are the problems?"
> and all. He tried to find and bring in problems, asking me if I
> had any sexual problems, any adjustment problems. I hones-
> tly couldn't bring any out. I felt adjusted to my pain. . . . He
> was definitely disappointed that I was normal. I actually told
> him I was sorry I was normal.

Just as the psychologist may expect chronic pain to lead to
personality disorder, he or she may expect all interpersonal
problems to be in some way related to the pain. Many pain
center patients object to this way of thinking because they
don't feel that the pain is *that* influential in their lives. In contrast, pain center patients do not feel that their interviews
with medical social workers are nearly as discrediting to the
self. The medical social worker may assert that there are
problems present in relationships with others but does not
assume that there are inherent psychological/personality
problems *within* the patient. In other words, the patients do
not get a sense of being blamed for their troubles by medical
social workers. In any event, patients are so desperate for
help at this point in their careers that they put up with these

clinical absurdities, although disagreement over the meaning of the psychological testing is often the genesis of later
conflict between the patient and staff.

The daily regimen of activities is highly structured. The
idea is to keep the patient as busy as possible in order to distract the patient's attention from the pain and to teach the
patient that he or she can actually perform at a high level of
endurance, at least compared to the usual inactivity. Each
patient receives a schedule of activities to follow. These
general activities may include vocational counseling, group
and individual exercise, swimming, and individual pain
therapies such as biofeedback, autogenic training, and (in
some centers) acupuncture. A crucial element of the operant
conditioning program is the systematic reduction of analgesic
drug use. Physicians normally prescribe these drugs on a
"p.r.n." (i.e., take as needed) basis, which can lead to erratic
use and abuse. Most pain centers enforce the following rules
in this regard: (1) no injections of any drugs and (2) an
accurate count of all medications taken in the center. Instead,
patients receive what Fordyce (1976: 157) and others refer
to as "pain cocktails." Briefly, a pain cocktail is a mixture of
cherry syrup and an pain drug. It is administered regularly,
say, one every four hours. Over time, the amount of drug is
reduced until the patient receives mostly plain syrup. This
programming eliminates the habit of taking large dosages
when the pain is most severe, yet still maintains control over
the intensity of the pain.

In addition to analgesic drug control, the operant program
tries to eliminate what are referred to as "bad" pain behaviors
and to reinforce "good" pain behaviors (see Fordyce, 1976:
103-119). The staff is instructed not to display sympathy or
extensive attention to complaining patients, thus reducing
their dependency. Activities such as work and exercise are
individually scheduled so that patients rest before the onset
of intolerable pain, in effect, increasing tolerance to pain.
The medical social worker counsels family members to stop

reinforcing bad pain behaviors of sympathy. Patients are forbidden to tell each other about their pain problems in order to teach the patients that their pain should be their own burden and responsibility in life.

In some centers, the patient actually signs a "treatment contract" on admission to the program (see also Sternbach, 1974: 94-99). The treatment contract, which is usually designed specifically for each patient, lists the responsibilities of the patient as well as the staff. The patient, for example, may promise to work hard to reduce the pain, to want to return to work, to improve the accomplishment of duties within the family, and so forth. The staff promise to help the patient achieve these goals but never promise to eliminate all pain. The underlying principle here is to return responsibility for pain and its management to the patient who has, at this point in the career, placed all responsibility for suffering in the hands of health care workers.

Patients' experience of and reaction to the operant program, again, varies according to the staff's perceptions of "good" and "bad" patients. Good patients follow the schedule closely, try hard to improve their work and exercise endurance, and so on. The bad patients tend to complain frequently about the rigid structure of the program, the impersonal style of the staff, and the like. Many patients change from being good to bad during the course of their stay at the center as their prior expectations of a potential cure are shattered:

> I thought I had a good attitude when the whole thing started. I wanted to cooperate. But things turned sour when I finally realized that they really weren't doing anything for the pain. All we did was mostly a lot of group talk stuff and exercise. . . . I didn't go there just to be told I was weird.

Most patients appear to respond well to the specific activities in their schedules. They learn that their tolerance for pain is higher than they previously imagined. For inactive and socially isolated patients, a simple card game or group wood-working project reminds them of the rewards of sociability. The most positive response is given to the therapeutic treatments that actually help *reduce* the pain, as would be expected. These instrumental elements of the program come closest to matching the patients' expectations. Surprisingly, most patients respond well to the pain cocktail idea. They enjoy learning how to lessen their dependence on debilitating and expensive drugs.

Most patient disappointment centers around the psychological/counseling encounters with the staff. They often feel that they are being blamed for a physical malady that they perceive as being out of their control.

> I really got fed up with hearing all the time that I don't react well to my pain. What do you expect, martyrdom? The shrink [clinical psychologist] told me I was way too dependent upon others for help. What a joke! So what if I ask my wife to take out the garbage when my back acts up? She wants me to do things for her all the time. . . . That's part of being married, I guess.

In order to understand why some pain center patients are more cooperative than others, we must bracket the unrealistic notion that bad patients simply do not want to be rid of their pain because they receive too many interactive and emotional benefits from it (see Sternbach, 1974: 55-77). The patient's experience in the pain center program is much more complex than that. Method of payment, for example, is an important indicator of patient attitudes. Good patients tend to be those who pay their own way. Since the program is so expensive, these patients try to get as much out of the center as possible. This high level of personal motivation leads to an openness to the staff's definition of the situation. Good patients are less likely to dissent openly from the staff's professional opinions. Much of the good patients' positive attitude and cooperative identity is, however, frontwork designed to mask occasional feelings of conflict and frustration. This frontwork is part and parcel of projecting the identity of a *competent* pain center patient. The good patients' past experiences have taught them that *health care workers are more efficient and put more effort into their work when patients are perceived as well motivated and cooperative* (see Fagerhaugh and Strauss, 1977: 122).

Bad patients tend to be those whose presence in the program is not of their own making. They agree to enter the program as a condition for maintenance of disabled status. In other words, their insurance companies, trade unions, or employers request (or even demand) that they *do something* to try to get better and return to work. Since these patients are not paying for the program out of their own pockets, their motivation for obtaining maximum benefit from the program is relatively low. The staff's opinion that bad patients do not really want to get rid of their pain is patently absurd. All pain-afflicted people categorically want to be rid of their pain. The bad patients have simply learned that the *identity* of being a pain-afflicted person accrues certain material benefits that, from their perspective, help compensate for their suffering. Thus many bad patients consciously try to appear uncooperative and refuse to present amenable frontworks because they want to reinforce their pain-ridden identities. They don't want to take the chance of having cooperation confused with a staff evaluation of: "He's not complaining, so he can't be hurting *too* badly."

These experiential characteristics of good and bad patients are, of course, somewhat oversimplified. There are some bad patients who pay their own way and later become disillusioned, as well as good patients who are present in the center due to work-related injury. Neverless, this analysis of the pain center experience strongly suggests that *successful patients may be more self-selected than shaped that way by the operant conditioning program,* in those centers that stress this particiular modality. Some centers acknowledge

implicitly this process of self-selection by awarding certificates of completion to their patients (see Sternbach, 1974:
106-107). The so-called good patients receive "pain expert"
certificates indicating that they have followed all the rules
and have tried hard to succeed. The so-called bad patients
receive "perpetual pain patient" certificates indicating that
they have either questioned or engaged in conflict with the
rules and the staff. These certificates are usually awarded
during the final group meeting of the cohort. This practice of
publicly shaming bad patients indicates a severe gap between operant conditioning theory and practice. It should be
recalled that operant conditioning is a process of changing
externally observable behaviors by programmed manipulation of the environment in which the behaviors occur
(Fordyce, 1976: 74-82). It is argued that the subject's behavior can be changed without recourse to the subject's conscious decision making. If these pain center staffs were
consistent in their espousal of operant conditioning, they
wouldn't blame the patient for his or her failure, but would
blame themselves and their programs.[21]

Objective evaluation of the effectiveness of the pain center
program is beyond the scope of this study. Researchers have
only recently begun to conduct long-term follow-up surveys
of patients who have completed their programs (Kotarba,
1981). This research, in general, shows that the effectiveness of the pain center regimen—in terms of reducing drug
dependency, increasing the patient's daily activity level, and
returning the patients to productive work—diminishes greatly
over time, especially for those programs that practice operant
conditioning. One clue to understanding this ineffectiveness
comes from viewing the pain center as a controlled, laboratory setting. Recent research in cognitive psychology strongly
indicates that laboratory learning occurs under different sets
of rules than learning that takes place in the real, everyday
world (Houston, 1976: 92-93), so that the behaviors and
attitudes learned in the pain center may be irrelevant to nor-

mal life. While in the center the patient is responsible solely
for being a good patient and can focus all attention on this
expectation. In everyday life, however, the patient must
mediate a range of personal and social responsibilities, of
which pain management is only one. For example, Dorothy,
a 32-year-old housewife, explains how changes in the con-
texts in which pain is experienced relates to "backsliding:"

> It's really easy to feel good about your pain when you're
> locked up in the clinic. You don't have much time to think
> about it because they keep you so damn busy all the time.
> Don't kid yourself . . . but the exercises aren't too bad at all.
> You pretty much set your own pace. . . . I don't think they
> understand how much things change when you go back home.
> I still gotta chase the kids around and pick up after them. My
> husband still expects dinner ready when he gets home. . . . I
> can't get through a day like that without a Darvon or two
> (laugh) or three. I'd go crazy.

In a sense, then, the pain center experience for Dorothy, as
well as for many other pain-afflicted people, is a *vacation*
(albeit an expensive one) or respite from the everyday
drudgery of mothering and wifing and working while in constant physical discomfort.

During the course of this research, I interviewed 29 former
pain center patients, including 5 who dropped out from the
programs before completion. I found that their retrospective
evaluations of the programs were mixed. In general, those
patients who experienced a humanistically oriented program were grateful for the concern and empathy afforded
them by the staff, as opposed to those patients who experienced a behaviorally oriented program and felt that they
were personally blamed for their problems. Most of my subjects indicated varying degrees of backsliding, even those
who were evaluated by the staff as successful. In general,
these patients felt that the pain center program is useful for
learning how to control drug use and how to maximize levels

of activity, but they firmly concluded that their pain center experience did not mark the end of their search for meaning for suffering. The pain center is rarely the last benchmark in a chronic pain career because it is not designed specifically to provide total pain relief, every pain-afflicted person's ultimate goal.

WHY COMPLEMENTARY HEALTH CARE MODALITIES?

I have shown how CHCM become viable alternatives to normal medicine when the direct intervention of physicians is perceived as ineffective. There is one other causal dimension, so to speak, to this phenomenon that deserves some discussion. Veteran pain-afflicted people, over time, reflect on the search-for-a-cure process itself. They try to make sense of their doctor hopping and their involvement with bizarre interventions. After a series of failures in the search, pain-afflicted people construct *secondary* reasons or accounts for trying something new. These secondary reasons help them to lower what are now perceived as unrealistically high expectations and to be prepared for other possible failures encountered before ultimately finding a cure.

In lieu of an actual cure, CHCM provide the means for avoiding current medical offerings while maintaining hope for *future* medical success with chronic pain. Many pain-afflicted people, as well as members of the general population, harbor intense fears of surgery and drugs, medicine's current response to pain. CHCM are ways of avoiding medicine until it develops a safe and effective way of treating pain. In the interim, CHCM provide a safe way of easing the guilt that emerges when the pain-afflicted person realizes that he or she should be doing *something* about the pain. As an illustration, several participants in a local YMCA "Healthy Back" exercise class felt this way. These participants, all middle- and upper-middle-class housewives, bounced around from one type of YMCA course to another (e.g., yoga, aerobic dancing, and swimnastics) in the attempt to do something about their chronic pain. They would try the first course, enjoy it, but later realize that they were either too busy or too lazy to continue the regimen at home without the support of a classroom environment. After awhile, they began feeling guilty and would then sign up for yet another related course, and so on.

CHCM, with the exception of pain centers, provide relatively inexpensive pain care compared to medicine. Over the course of a lengthy pain career, this economic factor may become quite relevant to an individual who perceives the need for constant health care.

Finally, we should note the social class differences in CHCM utilization. It is now clear that, contrary to the traditional sociological literature, which views CHCM as essentially lower- or working-class options, members of all socioeconomic class groups consult CHCM when needed. Social class does, however, partially determine *which* CHCM one may consult. Lower- and working-class pain-afflicted people are more inclined toward chiropractic, naturapathy, and faith healing for two reasons. First, they are the least expensive of the CHCM. Second, they may fit certain lower- and working-class notions of *proper* alternative health care (see Koos, 1954). Acupuncture, meditation, biofeedback, and hypnotism are more within the realm of the middle class for the same economic and cultural reasons. These modalities are relatively expensive and are rarely covered by personal health insurance. But there is a fascinating link between the use of these modalities and middle-class notions of proper health care. The American middle class is the bastion of the holistic health and self-actualization movements (Satin, 1978). For the sophisticated, middle-class patient, the use of holistic CHCM can contribute greatly to the sense of self-esteem by projecting the image of a person who is sufficiently creative to be knowedgeable of and inclined toward experimenting with innovative forms of health care.

NOTES

1. There is a fairly extensive literature in medical antropology on nonmedical healing. These studies are, however, normally conducted on non-Western, preindustrialized societies, thus limiting their relevance to the present study. Landy (1977) is perhaps the most up-to-date and comprehensive collection of such studies. Landy (1977: 11) insightfully notes the tendency toward convergence between the methods of medical anthropology and medical sociology:

> The differences are perhaps sharpest, it seems to me, . . . in the more holistic view of medical anthropology, its constant awareness of cultural context as a point of reference for everything that comes under its scrutiny, and for the participant-observer technique of the anthropologist as contrasted with the more particularistic, less personal, less intimate, and generally more formalized techniques of the sociological investigator. Even these distinctions today are more in tendency than in actuality, and it is no longer rare for a sociologist to become a participant observer and for the anthropologist to use the formal, systematic, quantitative techniques of the sociologist—each using these in addition to, rather than as substitutes for, his own traditional approaches.

The present study is designed to follow this convergence in style.

2. Wallis and Morley (1976) have edited an interesting collection of essays on various unorthodox forms of medical treatment. These essays, largely based on secondary sources of data, focus on the use of these modalities in England.

3. There are some fascinating works on quackery, always in defense of medicine and occasionally sponsored by organized medicine. Reed (1932) is a classic in this area. Smith (1969) is an especially biting condemnation of chiropractic.

4. See Douglas (1976: 55-82) for other techniques for piercing the veil of evasion, misinformation, and lies that often confront the field researcher.

5. This experience is quite similar to the naturapathic encounter. Naturapathy and chiropractic are almost identical healing arts. Members of both groups are often trained at the same schools, occasionally study both fields simultaneously, and utilize essentially the same therapeutic techniques (see Wardwell, 1978: 8-9).

6. Cowie and Roebuck (1975: 123-27) found that the chiropractor they studied relied heavily on personal referrals for new patients.

7. Like most chiropractic literature available in the waiting area, this brochure does not list any publication information.

8. In some states, chiropractors *must* use the word "analysis" because they are forbidden by law to diagnose.

9. In their movement toward professionalization, many chiropractors, especially younger members, have adopted the trappings of their medical competitors, like wearing white smocks. Some chiropractors have even begun to incorporate various kinds of modalities into their work, such as ultrasound therapy and acupuncture.

10. Since 1973, three new colleges of chiropractic have opened in the United States. Since 1972, chiropractic services have been granted limited coverage in both the Medicaid and Medicare programs (see Wardwell, 1978: 14-15).

11. There have been numerous words used to describe the object of mystical experience. Hindu yogas refer to it as the Godhead. Ethnomethodologists refer to it as Being (see Mehan and Wood, 1975: 172-173).

12. "Pain Can Sometimes Be Blessing From God." Billy Graham's Answer, as appeared in the San Diego Union (April 21, 1979).

13. The German Idealist tradition, which has been reflected in the Transcendentalist Movement in the United States, is a secular form of ascetic literature, philosophy, and methaphysics (see Lovejoy, 1961).

14. This is a pseudonym for a small, state-supported university on the West Coast.

15. I obtained this information from an examination of informal information sheets completed by all students. The class instructor gave me permission to see them. Otherwise, I was simply another student in the class and was able to engage in unstructured conversations with other students as such.

16. There are several variations of acupuncture that do not require the insertion of needles. Moxibustion is the burning of a mosslike derivative of the mugwort plant. It is placed upon the body point where needles would otherwise be inserted. Indigenous acupuncturists argue that the heat from the burning moxa has the ability to draw out excessive energy from the body. Acupressure is the technique of massaging the body point (see Kotarba, 1975: 172).

17. This estimate is derived from an analysis of the *Pain Clinic Directory* published by the American Society of Anesthesiologists.

18. Data for this analysis were obtained through my own observation of and participation in various pain center activities, observations of various professional meetings such as the annual Colorado Pain Symposium, and an examination of the professional literature.

19. The six months duration of pain criterion seems to be modeled after legal and risk management criteria.

20. Some pain center costs are covered by private or group health insurance, but this kind of coverage is still quite uncommon. Some carriers insist on paying only for specific services delivered during one's stay in the pain center. For this reason, many centers have established outpatient services.

21. Haney and Colson (1980) discuss the ethical implications of a physician's assessment of "good" and "bad" patients. They conclude that an effective and ethical encounter can exist only when the physician and patient agree on the basic value assumptions informing their relationship, and when the physician controls for his or her own value biases by being concerned only with what is functional for the patient.

5

"PLAY WITH PAIN, TALK INJURY": THE PROFESSIONAL ATHLETE

Secrecy is an essential property of the chronic pain experience. We cannot perceive another's pain as easily as we could a broken limb, paralysis, or the advanced stages of cancer. Pain-afflicted people appear quite normal in the absence of other illnesses or physical disabilities. We cannot see lower back pain or a migraine headache. We might expect certain elderly people to be in pain due to the aging process, but we certainly do not expect a young and otherwise healthy-looking person to be experiencing protracted pain with little hope for a cure.

Without any observable physiological evidence that indicates a person may be in pain, we can only know of another's suffering through the communication of the *idea* of pain. The notion that we can construct intersubjective understanding of physical sensations like pain has long been the subject of philosophical discussion. Wittgenstein (1953: 244-246), for example, used pain to illustrate his argument that words for sensations are used *in place of* the behavior that is the natural expression of the sensation; they do not refer to the pain. Words are simply new pain behaviors. The verbal utterances and their corresponding natural pain behaviors (e.g., "I hurt" as opposed to crying and groaning) are both *incorrigible propositions.* Wittgenstein argues that a person cannot be in error as to whether he or she is in pain. Furthermore, one cannot logically *doubt* the veracity of another's declaration of pain. We can be victims only of false ideas, not of false sensations. Another's verbal expression of pain makes sense to us primarily because the words are part of a common language and only secondarily because we can relate the words to our own, private experiences of pain.[1]

This type of philosophical/linguistic analysis lays the groundwork for understanding how it is possible for us to talk meaningfully about nonvisible pain. When we observe the actual empirical situations in which chronic pain emerges as conversationally relevant, however, we see that pain talk is highly problematic in form and situational in use. Certain audiences may in fact doubt the veracity of pain statements. The pain-afflicted person may be discredited if the audience at hand has reason to believe that the speaker is falsely claiming pain in order to be relieved of unbearable role expectations or to obtain secondary benefits. This is the rationale underlying the imposition of the label "malingerer" (see also Szasz, 1956).[2] Even if the audience agrees that the speaker may in fact be in pain, it can accuse the speaker of verbally displaying a more agonizing level of suffering than actually exists.

The pain-afflicted person may decide to conceal the experience of pain from potentially critical audiences if the social and emotional costs resulting from disclosure far outweigh the perceived benefits. The benefits of pain disclosure include access to health care, sympathy for one's suffering, and help in adjusting to everyday contingencies affected by the pain. But the costs of pain disclosure, as learned through experience, can be perceived as overwhelming. Certain reactions of critical audiences may elicit feelings of shame and guilt.

The pain-afflicted person feels shame on learning that his or her embodied identity is judged to be defective or incapacitated. Likewise, a feeling of guilt results from the sense that One is somehow held responsible for one's suffering, as would occur when one's pain emanates from a fall incurred while being drunk. A more practical consideration, though, is the potential material cost of pain disclosure. If a high level of physical competence is a requisite for one's job, pain disclosure can threaten job security due to its commonsense identification with injury or disease.

Situations in which pain disclosure decisions have to be made permeate the lives of pain-afflicted people. We need only to look at the nature of the affliction to understand why. Since chronic pain is in most cases a fairly constant if benign experience of discomfort, it accompanies the individual in all social situations. But chronic pain is rarely sufficiently serious to warrant designation as a "primary relevance" (Schultz, 1964: 125). Chronic pain is relevant when it is the focal point of interaction. This occurs when the pain is initially defined as acute, when it is the topic of interaction with health care workers, or when it overtly hinders the social task at hand. At most times, though, chronic pain is an *experiential context* for other role-determined, everyday activities. Chronic pain modifies these social endeavors. Thus the pain-afflicted person exercises a certain amount of control over the intrusion of the pain into social interaction.

Observable chronic pain behaviors are best conceived as *situationally elicited.* Psychological and anthropological literature that argues that pain behavior can be explained solely by either personality (e.g., Petrie, 1967) or cultural types (e.g., Zborowski, 1969) is only partially correct. These arguments are based on observations made in highly con-

trolled situations (e.g., personality inventory tests) and settings (e.g., hospital wards). When we observe varied natural
settings in which chronic pain is socially actualized, we find
that there are very few pure stoics and stentorians. The pain-
afflicted person who is critical and demanding in the orthopedic ward in order to get desired assistance from the staff
may be quite secretive about the pain at home or at work,
where talk of pain could be seen as totally counterproductive
and disruptive.

Professional athletes are excellent subjects for the study
of situated pain behavior. The nature of their work demands
extremely high levels of physical competence.[3] Incapacitating injury or the threat of injury such as that posed by chronic
pain can bring an athletic career to an abrupt halt. Moreover,
the violent nature of many professional sports leaves participants susceptible to career-damaging injury. Injury and
pain have intrinsic, primary relevance to professional
athletes, if not during the distracting frenzy of the game, then
during routine visits to the team trainer.

In the remainder of this chapter, I will discuss the ways
professional athletes manage chronic pain within the general
context of athletic injury. The focus will be on baseball, basketball, and football—the dominant forms of professional
sports in the United States.[4] I will use the experience of professional athletes to develop general principles underlying
the communication of chronic pain that can be applied to all
pain-afflicted people. In Chapter 6, I will test these principles against the chronic pain experiences of blue-collar,
manual laborers who are also dependent on high levels of
physical ability for continued job success, but who in general
demonstrate less motivation for concealing chronic pain
from their critical audiences. In both chapters, I will em-
phasize the importance of occupational subcultures in developing communication strategies.

It should be noted that the work-related health care available to both groups of workers falls under the general rubric

of "occupational medicine." In Chapter 6, I will contrast the social organization of these two forms of occupational medicine in order to analyze their effectiveness in dealing with work-related chronic pain.

TALKING ABOUT PAIN

When athletes talk about work-related health problems, they often use the expression: "Play with pain, talk injury." On the surface, this expression appears to be just another addition to the body of jargon commonly known as "jock talk." But investigation into the subjective meaning underlying its usage reveals how it neatly summarizes the options a player has in deciding what to do about physical problems. Put simply, *play with pain* refers to the decision to prevent a physical problem from interfering either with one's athletic identity or with one's play. *Talk injury* refers to the decision to disclose a physical problem to potentially helpful (or discrediting) audiences such as coaches, trainers, management, the press, or the public. The variables that influence these decisions include visibility and severity of the injury, age, and the location of the problem in the athletic career continuum. The major factor influencing this decision, however, appears to be the athlete's perception of his or her job security.

We should note that athletic injuries are a normal and expected part of the game (see Edwards, 1973:325-328). It is very unusual for any professional athlete to complete a season without some sort of injury. In his survey of injuries in the National Football League, Underwood's (1978: 72, 82) found that in 1977 there was a 100 percent casualty rate (i.e., one injury for every player) and twenty quarterbacks incapacitated by injury. The dramatic fall of the New York Yankees and Los Angeles Dodgers in 1979 can be at least partially attributed to the rash of injuries to their pitching staffs. An underlying principle in professional sports is that while injuries are to be expected, their disruptive effect will be minimized by getting injured players back in shape as quickly as possible. One National League trainer told me that in the course of a season he will work on *every* team member at least two or three times for some type of injury.

Observable, disabling injuries are the most commonly perceived and talked about injuries in professional sports. Examples of this type of injury include shoulder separations, fractured limbs, and concussions. Reactions to these injuries are fairly unproblematic because both the injured athlete and critical audiences are aware that these injuries are serious, occasionally life threatening, and definitely incapacitating. An athlete would find it very difficult to conceal an injury that places him in a hospital's intensive care unit, which of course he would not want to do. Since these types of injuries must be attended to immediately, they need not concern us in the present study.

Player reaction to *nonobservable, restricting injuries* is somewhat more problematic. The most notable example of this type of injury is the muscle pull. A muscle pull (or strain) is "damage to a muscle or tendon occasioned by overuse or overstress" (Encyclopedia of Sports Sciences and Medicine, 1971: 76). Muscle pulls vary in seriousness, but a large proportion of them can be concealed yet still be painful. In other words, a player may be able to play with a muscle pull without limping, restricting throwing movement, or even reducing running speed and mobility. The player's perception of his athletic identity largely determines to what degree he will allow the injury to limit his playing time and whether or not he will disclose the injury to others. Players with *secure athletic identities* (SAI) tend to reveal such injuries and use them as justifiable reasons for excusing themselves from play. SAI players are those who are of "star" caliber and/or who are protected by long-term, no-cut contracts. The disclosure of a minor injury does not threaten the player's career. The player is so valuable that critical audiences can only hope that he heals properly and returns to the team as quickly as possible. Indeed, management may feel that they have too much invested in such a player to risk his permanent loss to the team by having him play hurt.

In this era of long-term, multimillion dollar contracts, many coaches and team executives are fearful that such job security can lead to malingering among their stars, as the following excerpt from the Associated Press (January 12, 1979) affirms:

> Walt Frazier, the Cleveland Cavaliers' inactive $400,000 guard, says a New York doctor has found a stress fracture in his foot, where Cleveland team physicians have found nothing.
>
> "I get tired of reading where I'm faking it," Walt groused. "I get tired of my foot hurting. They [Cavs physicians] take x-rays and they never find anything. It's like I'm telling a lie. Dr. [John] Marshall shot my foot full of dye and he found a stress fracture."
>
> But Cleveland Coach Bill Fitch said he checked out the injury differently, and gruffly replied to a suggestion that Frazier might never play again for Cleveland: "That's obvious, isn't it?"
>
> Fitch said he resents Frazier's remarks and defended the Cleveland doctors. "Our doctors are all-stars in the NBA. They are the best in the league. We called Dr. Marshall and he didn't say Frazier had a stress fracture. And our doctors didn't find any." Fitch added: "I know the foot is sore. Threshhold of pain is a mental thing. Some guys can play with pain."
>
> He didn't elaborate that, to him, Frazier cannot.

The SAI players, on the other hand, feel that long-term contracts protect them from management's traditional pressure to play at all (physical and emotional) costs. Don Drysdale,

the former star pitcher for the Los Angeles Dodgers, recalls
the shift in his attitude toward total dedication to the team:

> I was taking so many things [for a shoulder injury] that I was
> like a walking drugstore. The doctors didn't want to give it to
> me but I insisted on it because I wanted to keep going out
> there. Of course, we had to play to get paid. Now, with the
> multi-year and multi-million-dollar contracts, I might sit
> back and say, "Wait, I'm not going to play until this s.o.b. is
> well" [quoted in Maher, 1978: 7].

The most famous case of an SAI player refusing to play in
pain is that of Bill Walton, former star center of the Portland
Trailblazers basketball team. Walton refused to play when
he learned that high doses of painkillers he was instructed to
take and that allowed him to play hurt resulted in a stress
fracture in his left foot. It is Walton's famous case, in fact,
which has highlighted recent investigations into the excessive use of analgesics and anti-inflammatory agents by professional teams in order to keep their injured players active
(Mandell, 1976).

Players with *insecure athletic identities* (IAI) may find
good reason to conceal nonobservable, restricting injuries.
IAI players are those who perceive their job status as being
in constant jeopardy due to the high level of competition for
positions in professional sports. They may be unproven
rookies, aging veterans trying to "hang on," minority group
players who feel that their ethnicity places them at an inherent disadvantage in job competition, or simply average
players on year-to-year performance contracts. IAI players
feel that they cannot risk having the coaches or the management use a minor injury as an excuse for dropping them from
the team roster, in view of their other shortcomings. Rookies
and aging veterans are most concerned about avoiding the
devastating label "injury prone." This label refers to the
identity of being a poor physical risk for long-term team

investment. IAI players believe the imputation of this label can be beyond their own control.

For example, Tom and Frank are both rookies on a National League baseball team. They have become very close friends since spending several years together on the same minor league clubs. One day in the middle of the season, Tom had a minor accident at home and cut his finger. The lesion required several stitches, and Tom duly reported the accident to the team trainer as required by league rules. When the team manager learned of the accident, he "hit the roof." He refused to believe that it was a pure accident, insisting instead that Tom must have been drinking at the time or is just plain "clumsy." Tom was sent back to the minor leagues one month later. During the latter part of the season, Frank also cut a finger, but this lesion occurred during pregame warm-ups. Having learned from his close friend's bad experience, Frank did not notify the team of his injury but simply consulted a private physician, at his own cost, for assistance.

Tom and Frank's experience demonstrates how quickly a neophyte professional athlete learns to conceal certain injuries from critical audiences. Robby is a 24-year-old second baseman. During his rookie year, Robby pulled a hamstring muscle in his right leg while running out a ground ball. The injury was slow to heal, so the team sent Robby down to their Triple A (i.e., minor league) team for what they claimed was "giving me all the time I needed to get my leg back in shape." On arrival at his new team, Robby began hearing rumors to the effect that the owner thought he was injury prone and was, therefore, looking to make a trade for another second baseman. Robby then began faking a quick recovery and, with the help of muscle relaxants obtained through a private physician, was able to play once more at his previous level of competence. He is now back in the major leagues and performing on a leg that was never given a chance to heal properly.

Trent, a 35-year-old first baseman, is an example of an aging veteran fighting the injury-prone label. Trent has started at his position for eleven straight years and has done sufficiently well to be chosen for several All-Star games. As the years creep up on him, Trent realizes that minor pulls and strains heal much more slowly than in previous seasons. But Trent never mentions these aches and pains to his critical audiences because there is a promising rookie on the team ready to take over Trent's starting position as soon as Trent is designated "over the hill:"

> I gotta play every day now, whether I hurt or not. Dade [the general manager] has been on my ass ever since Kyler [the rookie] came on like a hot-shot in spring training. I just have to try and stay in better shape. If this club cuts me, I'm finished. Who's gonna pick up a thirty-five-year-old first baseman?

The fear of having one's athletic identity spoiled by injuries results in IAI players downplaying injuries. They rely extensively on the team trainer and physician to get them back on the field as quickly as possible. But excruciating pain is often reported as mild discomfort and stubborn injuries are often reported as healed long before they actually are. IAI players commonly claim that they can "shake off" most physical problems, often in cases in which the trainer of team physician insists that the injury will heal only with rest.

Chronic pain problems are rarely disclosed by either type of professional athlete. These problems include back disorders, joint degeneration due to arthritic conditions, postinjury discomforts, and all the aches and pains associated with the stress of athletics and the process of aging. These types of problems may not directly affect playing ability, but are indications to others that the player is perhaps reaching the end of his career. The ability to mask these problems from critical audiences is the clearest illustration of "playing with pain."

Surprisingly, SAI players rarely talk about their chronic pain problems. Although SAI players' careers are materially secure, their sense of self-esteem is a matter of ongoing maintenance. The rewards of professional sports extend well beyond financial remuneration. Pride, dedication to a team endeavor, the admiration of fans, and the respect of one's peers are among the many intangible reasons why professional athletes "play with pain" and risk their present and future health status in order to fulfill their childhood dreams of being a "star:"

> I'd be playing baseball for nothing, if nobody wanted to pay me. Ever since I was a kid, all I wanted to do was play ball. I never really thought about doing anything else, like wanting to be a doctor or something. . . . Everybody does when they're a kid. . . . We're the luckiest guys in the world. We can do what we dream about all our lives and make a lot of money besides.

The maintenance of self-esteem is probably the major factor keeping SAI players motivated to play their best. A large part of the status of being a star athlete is the attribution of a superman identity by one's admirers. To admit that one is hurting or that one's knees are giving out after years of stress and strain is to admit that the glow of stardom is diminished. SAI players become quite upset when confronted by newspaper stories describing them as "slowing down," "ready for part-time duty," or becoming best suited for designated hitter status because their speed and defensive skills have lapsed.

Specifically, critical awareness of chronic pain problems may result in two kinds of negative reactions: shame and guilt. The SAI player feels shame when his previously impeccable ability is now defined as impaired. Shame runs especially deep when it correlates with diminished playing skills. Having one's self disvalued in such a way can be devastating because the athlete has always been able to base his presentation of self on virility and youth. The emergence of aches and pains marks the movement to an entirely different and sometimes frightening status in life. It is the prospect of being shamed that leads many veteran athletes to give up the game:

> I promised myself a long time ago that I would quit this game when it became more hurt and pain than fun. There are too many guys, I think, who make fools out of themselves . . . by not knowing when to hang it up. If you play hard and are lucky enough to last a few years in the big leagues, then you should be man enough to know when to quit. . . . They forget that this is a young man's game. It's tough.

The SAI player feels guilt when he perceives his critical audiences as blaming *him* for pain problems. The player may be criticized for not getting himself into proper shape to play, for not taking proper care of injuries, and for playing foolishly beyond his prime years. Professional athletes with chronic pain problems, like others in the general population, try to resolve this guilt by reflecting on the past and trying to figure out what they did wrong to *cause* their nagging pain problems:

> You always wonder "Did I try to play too soon after the injury, did I follow the trainer's orders right?" You never really know. In my case, I probably did play on my bad knee way too soon. . . . Doc Hardy, if I remember right, told me to stay inactive for, let's see, oh, it must have been six or seven weeks. But six or seven weeks is half a season. It's now or never, baby.

Marginal, IAI players talk least about chronic pain problems. They feel that if they can bear the pain, it is best not to reveal it and take the chance of losing their jobs. A young athlete who learns early how to mask his pain successfully can often have a long and worthwhile playing career. Gus, a former professional basketball player, is currently a television announcer for a National Basketball Association team. When Gus was a senior in college, he hurt his back during a game. The team physician diagnosed the problem as a ruptured disc. Surgery was performed immediately, eliminating the severe sciatic pain, but Gus still felt considerable discomfort when exerting himself in any way. Since he had come so close to reaching his goal of playing professionally, Gus continued to play in spite of the residual pain. He worked hard at the exercise regimen that was part of the postoperative rehabilitation program. By strengthening his entire body, he reduced the risk of reinjury. But above all, he was able to present the identity of an athlete who had totally solved his physical problems. Gus did not tell *anyone* that he was still in pain:

> I didn't tell anybody my back still hurt, no kidding. I remember, I came back to play out the last three games, and then to the playoffs [NCAA tournament]. Before the injury, people told me I stood a good chance of going early in the draft. You know, this was a dream come true for me. I wasn't going to blow it. . . . After the game I thought I was going to die. My back felt like a brick wall. I'd jump right into the whirlpool and sit there for an hour or more. . . . But I only did it after everyone had gone from the gym.

Gus was drafted in the first round, having successfully convinced the professional scouts that he was totally fit. His professional career spanned eleven successful seasons. For a few years, the high intensity of play distracted Gus's attention from his pain. The agony, however, came after the game:

> After a while, I got to know what my limits were. I only started a few games as a pro—big deal, huh?—mostly coming off the bench. So I wasn't getting that much playing time. . . . I was never really pushed. . . . Well, you don't feel that much

pain during the game; your mind's on winning and doing well. After every game, it was the same old story: ice packs and whirlpools.

During Gus's fifth year in the professional ranks, his back pain became nearly unbearable. He considered quitting the game, but decided that he could stick it out for the money and his love for the game. He tried muscle relaxers, back braces, heat, rest, and cold *before* each game because: "I had to be ready to play immediately." When he heard that the team's management was considering dropping him, Gus decided to try something new: chiropractic. A friend of his from college suggested it. Gus found that the chiropractic adjustment worked much better than the orthopedic treatments he had been receiving from the team physician. At first, Gus did not tell anyone on the team that he was seeing a chiropractor; he was afraid that the coach would disapprove. But when he felt the mobility in his back slowly return, Gus spread the word among his teammates, some of whom had back problems of their own. To this day, Gus firmly believes that the chiropractor was solely responsible for extending his career. Toward the end of his playing career, Gus tried many of the new treatments emerging with the chronic pain phenomenon, such as acupuncture and biofeedback. None of them was as effective as chiropractic.

When I asked Gus to reflect on his basketball career, he said that he would definitely play basketball if he had to do it all over again. He feels quite fortunate to be able to control his back problems when so many athletic careers are curtailed prematurely due to health problems. Now, however, Gus must face the possibility of arthritis inflicting his damaged spine, a common ailment among ex-athletes (see Maher, 1978: 8).

Gus was able to enter professional basketball because he successfully masked a potentially discrediting chronic pain problem from critical audiences. As his career developed, though, and Gus demonstrated prowess on the court, his position on the team was secured, allowing him to reveal both his back problem and the unusual health care modalities he utilized. Gus allowed his impairment to merge with his total athletic identity only when his physical imperfections were adequately compensated for by his overall professional competence. A complementary form of athletically oriented, chronic pain experience displays a reversed order of events. The athlete in this situation begins his professional career with untainted athletic identity but later develops a chronic pain problem that is increasingly removed from critical attention. The process of becoming an IAI is fought.

Alex is a 34-year-old American League outfielder who is probably near the end of his brilliant playing career. I say "probably" because he has recently undergone surgery on his left Achilles tendon, placing him on the disabled list for the third season in a row. Alex began his baseball career on a sparkling note. He was voted a college All-American while playing for an NCAA championship team. He was perceived by all as having outstanding potential as a professional player. With a strong throwing arm, outstanding running speed, good power, a keen batting eye, attractive appearance, and an articulate command of the press, Alex had all the makings of a superstar. And for several seasons, Alex lived up to the high expectations placed on him. But in the middle of the 1977 season, Alex suffered a "freak" accident that was to mark the beginning of his experience of chronic pain:

> We were in Kansas City playing against the Royals. There was a long-drive hit and I dove in an attempt to catch the ball. That's how the injury had happened, diving on the Astroturf and landing in a somewhat downward position. There was a twist in the upper body and in the lower part of my extremities . . . in a torquing kind of situation compounded by the force of landing on the Astroturf which doesn't give.

Alex had to be carried off the field, twisted in agony, on a stretcher. His entire back was in spasm, "from the top of my rear end to the base of my neck." Several days of bedrest and mild doses of muscle relaxants put Alex back on his feet, but he knew he was injured and would have to work himself back into shape. X-rays were negative in contradiction to Alex's drastically restricted performance on and off the field:

I went out for about three months (the remainder of the season), playing sporadically, not really being able to perform really up to a 100% level. And, uh, I had problems doing a lot of things. Not being able to pick up the shoulder at home, not being able to drive to the ballpark while, as a thirty-five minute drive, some days I had to stop and take a walk. I also fly my own plane. . . . One time in particular I flew to Phoenix and had to come back commercially because I was not going to take a chance flying myself back because my back had started to bother me.

The 1977 season turned into a disaster for Alex. The team orthopedic physician could not "put his thumb on" the physiological cause of Alex's constant pain. At this point, however, Alex truly believed that the injury and pain were both transitory and, like a typical person in pain, assumed that it was simply a matter of time before he found the correct form of health care intervention. Alex felt much pressure, though, in getting back in shape in time for the following baseball season:

After three months of this, it was the type of situation where, uh, "what do you have to lose?" so I had heard through a relative of mine about a chiropractor in Van Nuys, California, that has in the past worked with Olympic athletes, a couple of whom I had known for a fact had had back problems of one nature or another. So, normally, it was like a two-month wait just to get into his office to see him. . . . I was able to contact him through a few other people [fellow athletes] and I had an appointment within three days. . . . I saw him every day for two weeks. . . . What we discovered was that, in diving for the ball, I had somehow pinched a nerve in my neck. . . . There was a small amount of manipulation used, but not a heavy tug and a pull. . . . He's also an applied kinesiologist, so he used a little acupressure, too.

In the off-season, Alex began the standard rehabilitation program. He followed closely the orthopedic's recommended exercises to restore muscle strength in the back, eliminated excess sugar in his diet, which he was told "tends to tear down muscles and make them weaker," and jogged as much as possible. After regaining some mobility in his back, Alex began the 1978 season with great optimism. His play during the month of April was indication of a miraculous "come back," but the renewed success was destined to be short lived. Alex found himself favoring his sore back in order to avoid reinjuring it and "getting into some awfully bad habits." This strategy placed undue stress on the other parts of his body, resulting in a series of secondary injuries, including the torn Achilles tendon.

As other injuries began to accumulate, Alex consciously reevaluated his back pain. Through the press and other players, Alex heard rumors to the effect that management felt that he was finished as a major leaguer and was becoming injury prone. Alex himself realized that he was not a "spring chicken" anymore. Alex responded by playing down his chronic health problem (his back) and shaping his athletic identity so that it could be spoiled only by the newer, more acute, and therefore curable injuries. Thus Alex played with constant yet concealed back pain for those few games he could in 1978 and 1979. While Alex's critical audiences assumed that his career was now threatened only by acute injury, Alex privately tried to keep his constant back pain hidden.

During that portion of Alex's career in which his back pain was a glaring feature of his athletic identity, he was literally

barraged with suggestions from concerned fans about folk
remedies he should try:

> [Acupuncture] was suggested by people who used to write in.
> You know, if you're a ballplayer who's playing in a large city
> such as Kansas City, I could have written a book on all the
> remedies that people were telling me. . . . Oh, anywhere from
> little old ladies who told me to take a pint of alcohol and dilute
> fifty aspirins in it. And then take that solution and apply it to
> the affected area. Well, that's fine if the affected area has a
> headache [laugh] and I'm sure it doesn't do any good for a
> backache [laugh].[5]

Needless to say, Alex did not seriously entertain many of the
suggestions offered by eager fans. He may in the future,
though, as his body ages prematurely because of all the
stress and strain of trying to play with pain.

Minority group athletes often sense that they have IAI due
to their ethnic backgrounds. Marginal athletes are especially
careful not to appear physically impaired if possible. Many
are fearful of anything that might curtail what they perceive
as their only path toward social and economic mobility.
Racist tendencies in professional baseball are (justifiably on
occasion) perceived as placing the black athlete at an inherent disadvantage in the rugged competition for jobs:

> When you got two guys of equal ability working for the same
> position, and one guy is white and the other guy is black, the
> white player wins all the time. The black ballplayer has to
> always hustle for a spot, just to make up for being black. Now,
> take me for example. I'm pegged as being slow. Now, you and
> I both know that there are a lot of white outfielders playing
> regularly who are slower than shit. Man, who's that guy on
> your team, yah, Richie Zisk. Boy, that guy runs like mud. . . .
> The man [the manager] thinks I'm lazy, but, man, everybody's
> not Lou Brock.

In light of these ethnic contingencies, we witness incredible levels of stoicism among some marginal black athletes.[6] For example, Frank is a second-string NBA guard who has played in the professional ranks for three years. During this time, Frank has had what his trainer describes as "incredible lower back pain." The coaches and fans cannot perceive this pain experience because Frank plays with reckless abandon and never complains publicly about his back. The trainer is the only member of the organization to know about the pain and even he is sworn to secrecy. In fact, Frank never consults the trainer anymore for assistance for fear of having someone notice him in the training room. So Frank consults a private physician and physical therapist for help. Frank, like other black athletes who are unsure of their jobs, avoids the possibility of having his chronic pain defined by critical audiences as "laziness" or "inability to take the pressure."

THE ATHLETIC SUBCULTURE

The professional athlete does not make the decision by himself whether to play in pain or not. He has need of certain information in addition to his own perceptions of discomfort, seriousness, and relative disability. Such information includes the experience of other athletes with similar problems, sources of health care other than that provided by management, and strategies for either presenting or concealing the impairment from critical audiences. A little sympathy, of course, never hurts. But the dissemination of this information must occur within a trusting and confidential context. The press, management, and even the fans, as critical audiences, may stigmatize the athlete if they learn that he is seeking advice for a health problem. The social network utilized by professional athletes to "make sense" of illness and injury problems in confidence is the *athletic sub-culture.*[7]

The athletic subculture is not synonymous with the lay-person's notion of the "world of professional sports," which includes all types of occupational and leisure roles related to sports. In other words, the athletic subculture is made up of the exclusive interaction networks of the athletes them-selves. The athletic subculture is distinctively characterized by an extremely high level of camaraderie.[8] Within their subculture, professional athletes are relatively free to bare their most private experiences, both on and off the field. In this respect, the athletic subculture resembles Simmel's (in Wolff, 1950: 345) notion of the "secret society." Simmel notes that the first internal relationship of a secret society in the *reciprocal trust* among its members. Trust is required because the *purpose* of secrecy in the first place is *protection* of the group as well as the individual member. Specifically, the athletic subculture is a "relatively secret society" (Sim-mel, in Wolff, 1950: 346) since the existence of the group is publicly known, but certain types of knowledge and activity occurring within the group remain secret. The element of secrecy among athletes that concerns us here is the true extent of their injuries and pain.

One need only walk into any professional sports locker room and begin talking about athletic injuries to learn the extent of secrecy among players. Any one player may divulge certain information about his own physical problems to a trusted listener, but he will rarely discuss another player's physical problems beyond what is already publicly known. Professional athletes respect each other's injury and pain experiences because they are such crucial determinants of athletic careers.

Since many professional athletes distrust the effective-ness of health care provided by management, they consult each other regarding alternative sources of help. For example,

Pete is a 30-year-old NFL quarterback who pulled a hamstring muscle in the third game of the season. The team trainer contended that Pete's injury would take from four to six weeks to heal and requested that Pete be placed on the disabled list. Pete, however, didn't think that the injury was *that* severe and, besides, wanted badly to play the next game. While discussing his injury with the other players, a teammate mentioned that he was effectively treated by an acupuncturist several years ago. Pete immediately arranged to visit the acupuncturist who was able to return Pete to the team in time for the following week's game.

The athletic subculture is a source of illicit pharmaceutical drugs. Players who decide to play with pain sometimes cut themselves off from the prescribed drugs ordinarily obtainable from the team physician. Playing with a pulled hamstring muscle, for example, can be very painful yet safe. If a player intends to mask his hamstring from management, he must obtain muscle relaxants and/or pain killers from another source. This source is often located outside of professional sports in either the illegal drug market or in lay medical circles. A player with good contacts with outside drug sources is among the most valuable members of the subculture.

Probably the most important information circulated among athletes pertains to methods for masking pain and returning to play as quickly as possible after an injury. Slight changes in batting stance may reduce pain and allow an injured baseball player to step back into the line up. Certain stretching exercises may provide a player with sufficient mobility to fake normal movement, especially in baseball, where physical movement during the game itself is fairly sporadic. But above all, an intimate peer can help an athlete diagnose a pain problem before he has to reveal it to the team trainer. This type of advice can help a player evaluate the severity of the problem and whether or not it could be expected to be "shaken off." This lay diagnosis is helpful when the injured player is fearful that the trainer tends to *overdiagnose* problems presented to him.

The communication networks that comprise the athletic subculture extend throughout the different professional sports. A player in one sport may seek the health care advice of a friend who plays another sport. Intermural athletic friendships commonly originate while the players are student athletes at the same high school or college. The advantage of confiding in a friend who plays a different sport is twofold. First, the player has access to indigenous medical knowledge that develops in other sports. This process, for example, largely explains the dissemination of information on the benefits of stretching exercises from football to baseball. Second, these intermural encounters are easily kept secret from the critical audiences in one's own sport. The player need not fear having a health-related locker room conversation overheard by an eavesdropping media reporter. Moreover, the player's membership in the athletic subculture extends beyond his actual playing career. As the stress and strain of a vigorous playing career catch up with the ex-athlete, the athletic subculture provides a ready source of advice for managing the physical problems of aging.

Jack is a 67-year-old assistant baseball coach. He fashioned an illustrious career that prepared him well to be a hitting instructor. When Jack was young, he injured his knee:

> Early in my career when I was, oh, like eighteen, nineteen years old, my second maybe third year in baseball, I hurt my knee real bad. It stiffened up on me real bad. Of course, in those days you didn't have the medical attention ballplayers have now. It took a long time to get well, but it didn't bother me much until, oh, forty years later.

Jack recalls the pressure felt by ballplayers in the past, before the modern era of long-term contracts, to play with pain:

> Back years ago, you almost had to play with pain. . . . If you showed any indication that you couldn't take a little pain, why, they didn't particularly want you on the ballclub. It was a little more of a rugged game, I think.

The years of wear and tear on his knee finally caught up with Jack. While coaching for another team in 1967, the knee pain became unbearable. Jack consulted the team's physician only to learn that arthritis had set in the damaged joint. A series of cortisone treatments provided little relief.

During the following year, while in Florida for spring training, Jack happened on an old teammate who was now a major league scout:

> This other scout, still a friend of mine, was real friendly with Sam Snead, the pro golfer . . . who was trying to get this copper bracelet in all the pro shops around the country. . . . A pro player by the name of Bert Yancy had arthritis and he put a bracelet on it and in like six months he's back on the tour again. So I said: "Well, I've tried everything else, give me one of those bracelets." And I stuck that thing on my arm and two weeks time I had no pain in my knee and haven't had any since.

Jack still wears his copper bracelet religiously and is able to play golf without much knee pain. His subcultural ties extended from baseball to golf, with subjectively effective results. But all is not well for a man who still thrives on athletic competition. When I asked him how his golf game is progressing, Jack replied: "Well, *it's* in pain [laugh]!"

THE ROLE OF THE ATHLETIC TRAINER

The role of the athletic trainer is crucial in the management of professional sports injuries. The stereotypical image of the trainer as an old, cigar-smoking masseur and locker room caddy couldn't be further from the truth. Today's trainer is young, well educated (usually in physical therapy, kinesiology, or physical education), and aware of the latest advances in sports medicine.[9] The trainer is responsible for keeping the players in top physical condition and getting the injured players back in shape as quickly as possible: The most successful teams are the best-conditioned teams.

Although the trainer is an employee of the team management, his sense of responsibility is directed toward both the management and the players. Baseball players often refer to trainers as the "twenty-sixth man on the roster," indicating their importance to players' careers. For the player who decides to conceal an injury or play with chronic pain, the trainer is especially important because he has the skills needed to keep that player active and productive. But a player in pain must first have total *trust* in the trainer before divulging a potentially career-damaging health problem to him.

The trainer, then, often finds himself in the precarious position of having to balance his responsibilities. Management expects the trainer to keep them abreast of the progress of all team injuries while the players expect the trainer to handle certain matters in confidence. Team trainers tend to handle such dilemmas according to individual merit, but in accord with one general rule: A team member should not be allowed to play with an injury or pain if there is any risk of further damage by playing. Athletic trainers are exceptionally conscientious in abiding by this ethical standard. The injuries that may be perceived as playable in baseball include minor muscle pulls, myostitis (an inflammation of muscle tissue), arthritis, minor sprains, and spinal problems. Player/trainer confidentiality may be constructed around these types of injuries. Players who decide to play with more serious types of injuries do not ordinarily divulge them to the trainer.

Rookie baseball players find it very difficult to develop trusting rapport with trainers. Baseball has traditionally maintained an unwritten rule to the effect that rookies are banned from the training room. In the days when trainers simply gave rub downs, their time was supposed to be spent exclusively on the veterans who needed this care most. If a rookie needed a rub down, he was stigmatized as not being of major league quality. One National League trainer recalls the following example of a rookie getting into trouble for getting caught in the training room:

> One [rookie] went out [during practice] and threw about one hundred double plays. His arm was stiff, so I said: "OK, listen you don't have a problem, it's just that you're tired and you strained it a little bit. . . . Come in and I'll work on it so you can go out there without that stiffness." Well, the coach got all over him. . . . He saw him in here and gave him some shit. . . . The coach said: "All right, you're out of the line-up." So now, the guy's petrified to come in here for anything.

Today, as training programs become increasingly oriented toward *preventive* care through exercise, young players appear to be getting increased access to the trainer's services and the trainer as confidant.

The marginal baseball player who decides to mask a playable affliction is in most need of the trainer's trust. Although he may need the trainer's help in getting prepared for the game, he can't allow management to learn of his pain for fear of getting cut from the roster. Players and trainers together construct strategies for concealing their interaction in such cases:

> We have one player that has contramalasia of the knee, which is very painful. . . . It's like a headache, you know, it's

there but it can't get any worse or hurt your play much. He also had a little nerve damage in his elbow. . . . I have two [training] rooms here. Before a game, he comes in and puts an icepack on his knee and an icepack on his elbow. He takes a book and reads back in a corner where the coaches can't find him. . . . It would give them an excuse not to play the guy. I never want to give them an excuse not to play a guy.

Older players are most affected by chronic pain problems, especially arthritis and spinal conditions. They try not to reveal the true extent of their problems even to the trainer, let alone management. The major obstacle to realistic evaluation of these injuries is pride:

They don't want to admit that it's over. They'll come in trying to get stuff taken care of. They don't respond as quick as the younger ones. They'll quit getting treatment, saying that the thing's cured, but it's really not and they go out and play in pain.

Tom is presently an assistant coach for the last baseball team he himself played on. He is the perfect example of a player whose reaction to an injury was to: "spit on it and play on it." Tom's former trainer, however, was acutely aware of Tom's athletic decline. In fact, the trainer maintains that he has never seen a player play with more pain than Tom:

Tom was getting into his twilight. He was having so much trouble. His feet were destroyed by playing on the hard surface. He still knew he could play, but he knew that he didn't have what it took to enjoy playing anymore, I think.

During Tom's final season, his health deteriorated rapidly:

There was a play at second base one time. The second baseman went to tag him, he tried to avoid the tag, and it looked like someone shot him with a rifle. Boy, was he hurting. He had his sore feet . . . his knees started to hurt, his groin started to hurt. His back was killing him. All the joints were hurting.

The trainer knew that Tom was too strong to be hurting only from torn-up muscles, so he finally convinced Tom to see a private physician for a diagnosis. Blood tests revealed that Tom was indeed suffering from the gout. Since Tom refused to give up either baseball or his heavy drinking, which were aggravating his condition, he somewhat playfully warned the trainer to keep his health problem a secret:

> He always told me: "If you ever tell the manager I'm hurting and he takes me out of the ballgame, I'm gonna kick your ass."

Tom finished off the season without having his secret discovered by his critical audiences. By the following spring, however, Tom finally realized that his playing days were over. This decision was made easier to take when Tom learned that he could stay on with the team as a coach.

Athletic trainers use much discretion in entering into collusion with players because of the problem of malingering. Trainers have their own typology of players that they use to differentiate motives for seeking training care: *gamers* and *nongamers*. A gamer is the player who puts 100 percent effort into his game. He'll only consult the trainer when he is really in pain, ignoring minor discomfort.

A nongamer is the player who complains about every little ache and pain. He is always blaming injuries for inept performances. The most common complaint offered by nongamers is back pain, which is, needless to say, the most difficult to disprove. Trainers shy away from nongamers because of simple time limitations, but also because of the trainers' responsibility to management to keep all players in playing shape. The nongamer, usually because of unbearable pressure to perform well, does not really want to play.

SECRECY AT HOME

As situations change, professional athletes' desire to talk about injuries and pain changes. As we have seen, the player who feels comfortable discussing pain with his peers or with the trainer may not even mention health problems to management or the press. When the game is over and the player returns home, he may find it difficult to talk about pain with his wife and family. Indeed, intimate others are occasionally perceived as potentially critical audiences to the impaired athletic identity.

To understand this phenomenon, we must realize that professional athletes maintain a general air of stoicism regarding their pain. To them, pain is a natural element of playing sports and accepting pain is a natural element of the professional athlete's role. A former NFL receiver describes this common attitude:

> I think professional athletes, in any contact sport, learn to live with a little bit of pain. If I didn't hurt on Sunday night or Monday morning, I would feel like I didn't do my job. . . . Ever since you're a kid, you learn that it doesn't do any good to cry everytime you get hit. If you want to play, you have to pay the price, you know, you have to decide if it's worth the pain and discomfort.

This stoic attitude provides only a *context,* though, for interaction with intimate others. As Strauss (1959: 144-147) notes, we try to maintain a sense of continuity in our identities in order to demonstrate to others that there is a certain unity and coherence in our life purposes and goals. Athletic identities are constructed on certain highly esteemed qualities such as strength, vitality, youthfulness, and durability. The athletic identity serves the professional player quite well through the early stages of his career, both on and off the field. When the professional athlete gets married, which is usually at or near the beginning of his career, he presents an identity to his wife that is probably at its peak. In a manner of speaking, their relationship is at least partially based upon his athletic prowess.

As that prowess begins to diminish with aging and the toils of the trade, the professional athlete may perceive his identity as threatened. He may begin to fear that he may no longer be the man that his wife married and still expects him to be. A common means of coping with deterioration of one's talents is to attempt to extend the continuity of the past identity. For this reason, many professional athletes do not talk about their nonvisible pain at home. They are afraid that their wives will not be able to adjust to the changes going on in their bodies.

The athletes' wives are usually quite perceptive of their husbands' pain. As one professional basketball player indicates: "The wives have an intuitive grasp of the situation. They always seem to know when to leave you alone." This intuition is the result of living with a player for a number of years and learning what the subtle clues indicating pain are. The most common clue is the silence after the game. One football player's wife realizes that silence means pain:

> When Bob gets home from a game and says absolutely nothing, you know there's something wrong. It's time to hide the kids; they always like to roughhouse with their father. You know, I've just stopped planning on going out or doing anything after a game, in the evening. Bob just gets so tired and crabby lately. . . . I let him work it out himself.

The common strategy for players' wives, then, is to cooperate in constructing the fiction of identity continuity with the past. Instead of directly confronting their husbands' experience of chronic pain and aging, the perceptive wives discreetly try to direct their husbands' thoughts toward constructive projection into the future, for example, by initiating discussion in the off-season regarding business investments. The less perceptive wives attempt to turn the process of identity transformation into a topic of discussion. The seeds of conflict are sown in this behavior, for professional athletes find it difficult to project to a point in the future when their self-image won't be that of a professional athlete. This conflict can lead to severe marital discord if it threatens the athlete's most essential sense of self-esteem.

When the athletes project into the future, they normally prefer to use the designation "retired athlete" rather than "ex-athlete." The practical wife respects this choice of nomenclature.

PROFESSIONAL SPORTS CAREERS
AND CHRONIC PAIN

In this chapter, I have discussed the chronic pain experience among professional athletes within the more general context of the athletic injury. I have purposefully avoided simply trying to isolate specific instances of chronic pain and basing my analysis on them because that strategy would have distorted the essence of professional sports. *Pain in all varieties is an inherent feature of professional sports.* Injuries and pain are the rule and not the exception. All professional football players, according to their trainers, suffer at least one major injury in the course of their careers. Several baseball trainers have noted that, at any one time, at least 90 percent of the team members play with some level of pain. Thus the difference between normal and chronic pain is blurred in many cases. Nevertheless, these facts point to the inherently *irrational* aspect of playing professional sports. Professional athletes must ignore the fact that their work results in great pain. They also tend to ignore the future implications of current injuries and the wear and tear to which they expose their bodies. From their perspective, their life-long goal has always been to play professionally some day, and their blind dedication to fulfilling this goal transcends obvious physical costs.

We must, therefore, be cautious of indiscriminately applying sociological models of work and occupations to professional athletes. These models tend to impute a high level of rationality to career decisions and movements, which may be true in the professions or bureaucratic occupations, but is certainly less true for the professional athlete. There are limits to the often proclaimed thesis that sport is a microcosm of American society (see Ball and Loy, 1975). Professional sports may share certain economic and ritualistic structures with other societal institutions, but the subjective nature of members' participation differs in crucial ways. For one, I have encountered amazingly few athletes who consider their play to be work or a job. They argue that they would still play the game even if they were not paid to do so. In regard to the present topic, we have seen how pain-afflicted people, as well as Americans in general, develop extensive health care industries for the purposes of eliminating pain from their existence. Professional athletes, on the contrary, actively confront pain in their chosen work. Professional sports, as an occupation, is perhaps best compared with that of the ancient warrior.

The primary usefulness of the professional athlete's chronic pain experience to our study lies in the generic process of deciding when and how to talk about one's pain problem. At this level of analysis, we will now compare two types of occupation that, on the surface, appear to be quite different: professional sports and blue-collar, manual labor.

NOTES

1. John Hund, a philospher of remarkable insight, first brought Wittgenstein's writings on verbal displays of pain to my attention.

2. Field (1957) documents the efforts taken by the government in the Soviet Union to combat widespread malingering resulting from the enormous pressures placed on the Soviet workers to increase productivity sharply.

3. This fact is most often ignored by those writers who treat sports as just another type of occupation, or who focus strictly on the economic aspect of professional athletics (see Gregory, 1956).

4. The shortcomings of my study are obvious. My research contact with women's professional sports has been minimal. I have also chosen to ignore professional golf, hockey, track, soccer, and others due to space and time limitations. Nevertheless, it appears that baseball, basketball, and football are representative of the process I analyze in this chapter.

5. Alex may be mistaken in this regard. There is clinical evidence that shows that the topical application of alcohol-based aspirin solutions can in fact reduce cutaneous pain.

6. Of course, today's black superstar can afford to be as lazy if not as arrogant as the white superstar due to the security of the long-term contract and the growing awareness of the black player's value to his team.

7. The concept "subculture" has, unfortunately, tended to be associated with deviant groups exclusively. As Irwin (1977) insightfully notes, subcultures emerge whenever there is a perceived need for alternative values and support systems within our complex society.

8. Of course, players often fight among themselves, both on and off the field, but normally feel constrained in talking about these episodes to outsiders such as the press.

9. Sports medicine is becoming a very popular form of applied medicine in the United States. Much of this interests come from the explosion of amateur sports participation, as exemplified by the jogging craze. *The Physician and Sportsmedicine* is a major source of information on this relatively new subject.

6

"PLAY WITH PAIN, TALK INJURY": THE BLUE-COLLAR MANUAL LABORER

If the expression "play with pain, talk injury" reflects the essential principles underlying the communication of chronic pain, it assumes the status of conceptual *metaphor*. The use of metaphor in explaining and understanding social phenomena has a long and rich tradition in sociology. When Robert Park informs us that "our great cities, as those who have studied them have learned, are full of junk, much of it human," we vividly imagine the hopeless plight of those people who have been virtually discarded by the advances of urban progress. Likewise, on hearing Charles Horton Cooley's famous expression "the looking-glass self" and picturing ourselves in front of a mirror, it is easy to understand how we appear as objects to others. Metaphor allows us to comprehend new ideas about social life by demonstrating how they fit cognitively (i.e., how they make sense) with our own experience and knowledge of the world.

"Methaphor can be understood as an illustrative device whereby a term for one level or frame of reference is used within a different level or frame" (Brown, 1977b: 78). According to Ricoeur (1977: 173-174), metaphor is effective when it clearly posits *resemblance* between both levels or frames. This resemblance, however, does not mean that we can literally *substitute* one image for another, for people are not literally junk. Instead, Ricoeur (1977: 212-213) goes on to explain metaphor as the intuitive experience of seeing one thing as we see another. In other words, metaphor allows us to use the language we construct to describe one phenomenon for the description of a newly "discovered" phenomenon for which we posit some similar trait.[1]

As described in the previous chapter, the expression "play with pain, talk injury" (PWP, TI) is frequently used by professional athletes to indicate a player's options in deciding what to do about injury and chronic pain. We can translate this into a conceptual statement that describes the more generic process by which *all* pain-afflicted people decide whether or not to project their suffering into the social realm of identities and interactions. PWP refers to the decision to keep one's chronic pain a secret and not allow it to interfere with the goals of the immediate social situation. TI refers to the decision to disclose one's chronic pain to a specific audience in order to obtain specific reactions. Thus PWP, TI, and the professional athletes' experiences of pain to which it refers becomes a colorful, "illustrative metaphor" (Brown, 1977b: 107-113) to help us understand more common chronic pain experiences. In this chapter, I will apply this metaphor to another, albeit less glamorous, individual, the blue-collar manual laborer, in order to see him as a worker whose occupational identity, like that of the professional athlete, may be threatened by the disclosure of chronic pain.

The typical blue-collar manual laborer works hard for a living. He may or may not have acquired specific skills such as machine operation. He is most likely a construction worker, but may also drive a truck, work on a loading dock, work in a factory, and the like. Remuneration for his work varies according to the skills he has acquired, seniority, whether he belongs to a union, and geographic location (i.e., lower wages in "right-to-work" states). His income probably ranges from $8,000 to $20,000 a year; he certainly is not getting rich through his work.

COMPARISONS AND CONTRASTS

In order to apply our metaphor meaningfully, we should note some of the important similarities and contrasts between the two types of workers. The most basic similarity is that both depend on relatively high levels of physical fitness to make a living. A construction worker does not last long on the job if he cannot lift heavy objects or work outside in the heat and cold. For reasons of socialization, physiological propensity, or sheer personal preference, both workers enjoy envigorating work and prefer working "with their hands and backs than pushing a pencil and holding up a desk" (see LeMasters, 1975: 20-25).

There are several crucial differences between the two. The average professional athlete's salary is considerably higher than his blue-collar counterpart's, although his working career is much shorter. For example, the average salary in professional baseball in 1981 was approximately $125,000, whereas the average playing career in baseball is only 4.75 years. Critical audiences also differ in scope. Whereas the blue-collar manual laborer may be responsible only to his foreman or supervisor, the professional athlete's work is scrutinized by coaches, scouts, management, press, and fans. Overall, the role of the professional athlete can be said to be much more glamorous, more highly esteemd in our culture, and much better rewarded. In addition, *types* of physical skills and capacities differ greatly.

Unlike the professional athlete, who is exposed to a wide range of injuries on the job, the blue-collar manual laborer is most susceptible to back problems (Finneson, 1977: 37). The manual laborer's job ordinarily does not involve violent contact with others or extensive running. His hard work is basically lifting and pushing, whether it be a shovel, bricks, or garbage cans. Both workers, however, are susceptible to the same maladies of aging.

The major difference between the two workers is the fact that the manual laborer has in general less reason to conceal nonvisible, chronic pain problems. There are two reasons for this. First, the manual laborer works in a fairly low status occupation. Few manual laborers dream of doing this sort of work when they are children, unlike many professional athletes. It is the kind of job many men take because they do not have the education or training for higher-prestige jobs. Thus a job-related injury does not destroy a childhood dream. If a worker is unhappy with his tedious job, he may perceive disability compensation as a welcomed alternative. Second, the rewards for job-related injury may be, relatively speaking, better for the manual laborer than for the professional athlete. If a professional athlete's career is ended by injury, he may have to forfeit a six-figure annual income and resort to a more common way of making a living. A manual laborer, on the other hand, may receive up to 80 percent of his normal income from disability compensation if his injury is determined to be job related.

A manual laborer may not perceive his own situation in such objective terms, however. The material benefits of disclosing chronic pain problems may either be irrelevant or secondary to the symbolic costs of disclosure. Like the professional athlete, the manual laborer may decide to conceal non-visible pain if disclosure threatens his self-esteem. A large part of a manual laborer's self-image and identity may come from his ability to do his job well. The work-related values that define self-esteem for the blue-collar manual laborer are actualized within his peer group and reflected in the traditional focus for the world of the working man: the blue-collar tavern. Unlike the professional athlete's subculture, which is located in the locker room, the blue-collar worker's subculture is most readily observed in the bar.[2]

THE TAVERN SUBCULTURE

The neighborhood tavern has become the object of considerable sociological interest in recent years. Sociologists have generally accepted the view of the public drinking place as a location for inconsequential adult "play" (see Huizinga, 1950). The tavern experience provides the drinker with a culturally accepted means of escape from the hectic responsibilities of everyday life (MacAndrew and Edgerton, 1969), while providing him with an assortment of inconsequential, "fun" activities such as shuffleboard, table pool, and flirtation (LeMasters, 1975: chap. 8). The trivial nature of the tavern experience is reflected in the conversations that take place there, for "bar talk is essentially small talk" (Cavan, 1966: 58).

In my previous research on tavern sociability (Kotarba, 1982), I noted how the blue-collar tavern provides the setting for serious and (to them) consequential interaction among the clientele. Unlike most other sociological studies of the public drinking place, I focused on those topics of conversation that may appear trivial to the sophisticated, middle-class sociologist, but are of primary relevance to the lives of the working class. Specifically, I described how the clientele regularly attempt to solve drinking/driving problems through the dissemination of strategies for avoiding the stigma associated with arrest for drunk driving (e.g., techniques for bribing traffic policemen and information on locating influential lawyers in case of arrest). Health-related topics of conversation are also quite common, since the threat of injury and disability is relevant to the maintenance of competent, productive identities.

The incidence of chronic pain among working-class men is probably considerably higher than that of the general population (Sternbach, 1974: 60). Harsh, physical labor leaves one susceptible over time to spinal problems and arthritic degeneration. The manual laborer faces the essentially same problem as does the professional athlete with chronic pain: There are certain critical audiences from which the pain problem should be either totally concealed or presented in certain favorable ways. Advice on whether to *play with pain or talk injury* can be obtained from intimate peers who face the same issues in their own lives.

The introduction of talk about one's pain problem into bar conversation is constrained by the informal rules of the setting. If all eyes in the bar are glued on the television set during an important baseball game, it is obvious that a customer will not interrupt with complaints about his sore back. The atmosphere within the tavern changes situationally, though, so that one can more easily talk about pain when the bar is quiet and the main activity is serious talk.

Pain talk is usually initiated humorously. To bring up one's pain in a serious tone would give the listener the impression that the problem is "with me" and not just "with my back." This is an important consideration because the manual laborer, like all other pain-afflicted people, must present an image of competency to his audiences in order to retain self-esteem. Competence is achieved by showing others that one is in control of the pain emotionally and is simply looking for *instrumental* assistance, although a little sympathy along the way is welcomed if not implicitly requested. The customer will try to objectify the pain and present an identity that is at once stoic and not in any way indicative of hypochondriasis, self-pity, or malingering. Humor is an efficient way of protecting the customer from these potentially negative evaluations.

For example, Frank, an iron worker by trade, walked into his regular tavern one afternoon on his way home from work. As he took a seat at the bar and order a drink, one of his friends was about to leave. As his friend passed him on the way out, Frank exclaimed within earshot of all: "Hey, Tom, are you leaving already? Look, as long as you are on your way home, why don't you take my ol' sacroiliac with you. It's not doing me any good lately!" Everyone at the bar, including Tom, laughed at Frank's little joke. But Frank successfully introduced his back problem into conversation and proceeded to talk to the bartender and three other customers for one-half hour about his slipped disc.

Pain-afflicted customers have different purposes at different times for talking about their pain. Among the most common is the desire for sympathy. The bartender, as would be expected, often serves this function. As Sternbach (1974: 56-59) and others have noted, family members frequently lose patience with a person who is constantly complaining about pain and who may be perceived as increasingly turning into emotional burden. Over time, the pain-afflicted person learns to say little if anything at home, if the reaction there is negative, and instead seeks comfort at the bar. One female bartender recounts her experience with such a customer:

> Bill used to come in here everyday after dinner. You never saw such a dejected guy. He always sat by himself, never bought a round. . . . I think he said he hurt his back at work, that's right, a couple years back. . . . I was the only person he'd talk to. It was funny, all he wanted to talk about was his back and how much it hurt. His wife must be a real bitch, accusing the guy of making it all up. . . . He was a sad case.

Sympathy and understanding are not automatically extended to any customer who seeks them. New customers are not given license to talk immediately about personal troubles like chronic pain; they are simply ignored. Regular customers who are disliked in general receive negative reactions to talking about their pain. Two middle-aged women were sitting together in a neighborhood bar when a third woman, Grace, entered. As usual, Grace was wearing a neck brace for what she claimed was a longstanding whiplash injury. I had already known that the two women disliked Grace because they talked about her as being a busy-body and a gossip. Their reaction to Grace in this situation, in largely inaudible talk, was predictable:

> Here comes the old busy-body! She thinks we'll all feel sorry for her just because she wears that girdle around her neck. The only thing wrong with her neck is what it's holdin' up!

One might assert that this is only an example of how petty two old women can be, but I have heard similar comments made by males about other males who were believed to be malingering.

Among the more important reasons for entering one's pain into tavern conversation is the search for medical folk knowledge. In this situation the tavern subculture provides what Freidson (1970: 292) refers to as the "lay referral system." At this point in their pain careers, however, manual laborers are *returning* to the lay referral system after the initial encounter with medicine has failed. Manual laborers are much like professional athletes in this regard. Both have very few options regarding the initial health care intervention into their pain problems. The professional athlete is expected to consult the team trainer or the team physician. The manual laborer is expected to consult the company physician, the company nurse, the union physician, or other practitioners under contract to the employer. Both workers normally do consult these practitioners because their services are free and because the workers protect themselves by having a work-related injury certified by company representatives.

The blue-collar manual laborer returns to the lay referral system when the original health care intervention has proven unsuccessful. Consultation with subcultural peers usually results in much talk on the merits of chiropractic, naturapathy, and other alternatives to medicine that "really know what to do with a bad back." Medical folk knowledge obtained in the tavern provides the pain-afflicted customer with social meanings that reinforce his ultimate hope for a cure and counteract the powerful meanings of medicine that are increasingly perceived as illegitimate.

Dan's experience is a good illustration of this point. He injured his back while working in the garden one Saturday morning. While visiting the neighborhood tavern one day, he discussed his problem with Craig, a construction worker who had had extensive contact with a wide range of medical specialists who had given him only partial relief. Dan was complaining that his family physician accused him of exaggerating his suffering because he could find no distinct cause for the pain. An orthopedic specialist insisted that Dan have an exploratory laminectomy, a fairly radical procedure that offers no promise of effectiveness. At this point in his career, Dan was so confused that he did not know whom to believe or what to do. Craig tried to relieve Dan's anxiety by recounting his own experience with doctors:

> Don't believe a word these guys tell you. Doctors will always tell you it's all in your head when they don't know themselves what's wrong. That's how they can charge you fifty bucks a throw and laugh all the way to the bank. . . . And whatever you do, don't let those quacks cut you open. I've heard of too many guys crippled by back surgery. Look, why don't you give my chiropractor a call. He's pretty good and cheap to boot. He can tell you all about doctors and why they're all fucked.

Craig's advice must have been convincing, for Dan took it and has never gone back to his old doctor for his back since.

Some manual laborers seek advice on how to conceal chronic pain from their employers. This type of interaction can occur in either of two situations. First, the worker may be afraid of losing his job if a precipitating injury is discovered. Workers not covered by union protection or those workers still in probation periods with new employers face this dilemma. Second, the worker may sense that an impaired physical identity may preclude him from getting a job promotion. Phil, a machinist, found himself in such a situation. He was up for promotion to assistant foreman, but needed to pass a physical examination first. Phil has had back pain for several years, but never told anyone at work about it. He consulted his good friends at the bar who gave him the following advoce:

(1) Be sure to jerk your knees if the doctor hits them with a little hammer.

(2) Take two or three muscle relaxers (which were later provided by one of the friends) the evening before you go in for the physical. These will give you a good night's sleep and make you more flexible in the morning.

(3) Don't mention anything about your back pain. Even if you are stiff during the exam, tell the doctor that nothing is actually hurting you.

(4) Don't tell the doctors that anyone in your family has had any kind of back trouble. They may become suspicious of you if you tell them this information.

Phil passed his physical and got the promotion. It is interesting to note how this set of subcultural strategies contrasts with the strategies used by potential Army recruits during the Vietnam War. In the latter situation, many inductees tried to subvert the medical screening process by feigning physical impairment in order to *avoid* military service.

When working-class bar drinkers actively seek to subvert corporate use of medicine as a way of controlling employees, these men function as a *deviant subculture.* The dominant value in this case is the employers' belief that they have the right to regulate their employees' career patterns by means of medical criteria for physical fitness. Workers often view these medical criteria as obstacles to their own success. The decision to deceive medical agents of corporate control is most commonly made when the worker believes that his real or potential physical impairments are either irrelevant to actual job performance or can be overcome by personal effort and dedication. Since chronic pain is essentially nonvisible and does not necessarily have to emerge during a company physical, it fits this scenario well.

PAIN CONTROL IN THE TAVERN SETTING

Among the regular tavern customers who suffer chronic pain, sympathy and advice are only occasionally sought. Very few will talk constantly about their pain because they soon learn that to do so gives them the incompetent identity of a "bore" or a "crybaby." Although the talk surrounding chronic pain is situational, the pain itself is constant. The tavern milieu provides several means for minimizing the discomfort. The prevailing atmosphere in blue-collar taverns is for the most part jovial and playful. This pleasant atmosphere can distract the pain-afflicted customer's attention from the pain and interrupt the course of the pain's becoming a constant, cognitive obsession (see Sternbach, 1974: 31-39).

But more important is the use of alcohol in the tavern as the *prerequisite* for tavern sociability. Most pain-afflicted customers use drinking more or less as a folk analgesic for their pain, both consciously and nonconsciously. Alcohol becomes a legitimate alternative to the prescribed analgesics that many customers dislike because of their debilitating side effects or because of subcultural denigration of drugs in general as "hippy stuff." Needless to say, there is little sophisticated understanding among manual laborers of the "drug" aspects of alcohol.

These men also harbor an amorphous fear of radical medical interventions like surgery. Wally the "G-Man," as this middle-aged garbage collector is affectionately known by his peers, comes into his favorite tavern everyday after work. The stress of lifting heavy objects all day can be easily observed, for Wally limps in with what appears to be a severe sciatic nerve pinch. Wally refuses to see a doctor for his problem because he is afraid he would be put on disability. (Wally is a true remnant of the traditional work ethic.) After several drinks, however, Wally literally feels no pain and can be seen dancing merrily around the juke box and pool table. For Wally, alcohol is an effective alternative to medicine.

Physicians have long aware been of the analgesic property of alcoholic beverages. A few drinks not only alleviate pain somewhat but may also relieve muscle spasms associated with arthritic and vertebral disc syndrones (Leake and Silverman, 1966: 89-90). The regular use of alcohol as an analgesic, though, has definite shortcomings. None of the pain-afflicted customers begins his tavern involvement in direct response to pain but increasingly integrates his pain experience into his ongoing tavern involvement. The specific use of alcohol for pain relief frequently results in alcohol abuse based upon both physiological and social factors. As Sternbach (1974: 92) and other experimentally oriented psychologists have noted, alcohol is a poor long-term analgesic because the body quickly develops tolerance to it. Indeed, the long-term use of alcohol may increase the perception of pain.

The customer views this phenomenon differently. He notices that, at first, drinking makes him feel better and assumes that increased amounts of alcohol are later required because the underlying pathology causing his pain is simply worsening on its own (e.g., the natural effects of aging on arthritic conditions). For some drinkers, the increased use of alcohol spirals along with increasing levels of pain until only a drunken blackout provides adequate relief. Social factors come into play for those literally disabled by their pain. A person on disability compensation, for example, has enormous amounts of time on his hands to accompany guaranteed financial allotments. If this person is already used to spending his leisure time in the tavern, he may find himself spending time there when out of work (see also LeMasters, 1975: 25-26). Heavy drinking usually accompanies depression over not being productive and busy. The problem of depression is accentuated when the individual realizes that he must drink alone during the day when his partners are all at work. This problem is common to members of all occupational groups who have never developed hobbies or other alternatives to leisure-time tavern involvement.

Clara is the "day" bartender at a typical blue-collar tavern. Many of her regular customers are unemployed manual laborers. She became very close to one young man who was in constant pain due to a work-related accident about six years ago and whom she witnessed becoming an alcoholic due to his pain. The following excerpt from my interview with Clara vividly portrays this tragic example of pain-related alcohol abuse:

I: Tell me about your friend.

R: Well, he used to come in here all the time. He had an accident and almost lost his leg. I wasn't sure half the time if he really did have all that much pain or what it was, but if he did, after two or three drinks, he would start to relax.

I: You said he almost lost a leg?

R: Almost.

I: Did he feel the pain in his bad leg?

R: Yes. It was bad; because they—it was almost to the point of gangrene was setting in. They sewed the leg back on, but there was no circulation there. And then when there was circulation, he had pain.

I: Did he come in here quite often?

R: Yes. All the time.

I: Did he drink because of his pain?

R: Yes.

I: Why do you think he became an alcoholic?

R: The pain. Well, and then he couldn't work. He was on disability, and he didn't have any close family. He really had nothing else to do. So it's usually better to be with somebody than to be alone.

I: Did he talk to you a lot about his pain?

R: Yes.

I: How did he talk about it?

R: He'd tell me that his leg was really hurting. And at times I could tell when it really, really was hurting because he—you could usually tell when he was drunk and when he wasn't and was hurting. And when he wasn't drunk and he'd get up to try to walk, he would, you know, stagger or fall, because there just wasn't the feeling there that should have been.

I: Was he seeing a doctor about his pain?

R: Oh, yes, he was always going.

I: Was he taking medication for the pain?

R: Yes, a lot of painkillers.

I.   Were they doing him any good?

R: No.

I: Did he tell you that drinking made his leg feel better?

R: Yes.

I: How did he say that?

R: He'd say "well, I need another one. My leg, it's going away."

I: Tell me more about him. Was he a married man?

R: No, but he was at one time. He was a young man. He was only thirty-two.

I: He is young.

R: He passed away.

I: From what?

R: They don't know. They first thought it was a cerebral hemorrhage.

I: He was still a young man, though.

R: But by that time, he was an alcoholic. There was no doubt about that.

I: How do you know that?

R: Well, I took him out to my place. My girls were gone and I needed some help taking care of my animals and stuff. And while he was there, I didn't buy him any booze and he didn't have any money to buy any. And yet I had him out there for two days, three days, and he actually got sick because he didn't have the alcohol.

I: Was he still in pain at that time?

R: No. He was just, he was going through DTs.

I: How long ago did he have his accident?

R: Five, six years ago.

I: Did he have pain all those years?

R: Yes, I think so.

SECRECY AT HOME: TALKING "FAKED" INJURY

In the previous chapter, I discussed athletic trainers' use of the expressions *gamer* and *nongamer* to describe those players who put 100 percent effort into the game and those who use every little ache and pain to account for inept performance on the field. There is a parallel phenomenon in the world of the blue-collar manual laborer. A manual laborer may actively *seek* the identity of a pain-afflicted person to account for his inept performance on the job. Ineptitude in this case reflects either the inability to cope with the physical/emotional demands of the job or the inability to satisfy the family's material/financial expectations. Chronic pain is a common "cover" for blue-collar malingerers because they know that a claim of chronic pain cannot be medically disproven. This valid bit of folk knowledge is often obtained through the tavern subculture.

It is important to note that blue-collar workers, as a group, are much more inclined to malingering than their counterparts in professional sports. Again, the basis for this difference lies in the distinct status difference between the two occupations: In general, the manual laborer has less to lose. If he does not strongly adhere to a naive work ethic, the manual laborer may feel that the world "owes" him more than the relatively low wages provided by his occupation. When faced with crisis at home or at work, his competence as breadwinner can be maintained by demonstrating that his occupational incompetence is not his fault, but is the result of unanticipated injury. The positive reward for a false claim is relatively lucrative disability compensation.

Workers in the bottled water industry make a fine study of the malingering phenomenon. Our case study is the Sunnyland Bottled Water Company. The average route drivers for Sunnyland make eighty to one hundred stops a day. At each stop, they must deliver one or more bottles of water that weigh 45 pounds each. Needless to say, this is very difficult work. Two out of every ten drivers are injured on the job each year. The most commonly claimed injury is back related.

When route drivers are injured, they are immediately eligible for disability compensation. By law, the company must pay them two-thirds of their income (tax free) for a maximum of two years. The average disability payment at Sunnyland is 1196 dollars a month. In addition, the company is liable for retraining expenses if the worker can't be placed in a less physically demanding position with the company. Occasionally, a lump-sum settlement is made for permanently disabled workers, which may approximate 20,000 dollars.

For some workers on disability compensation, this recourse is perceived as an attractive escape from personal pressures. Malingering takes two forms. First, a worker may completely fake a back injury and pain. Bill is an area manager for Sunnyland. During his many years with the company, beginning with driving himself, Bill has noticed a pattern of faked injuries:

> Their job starts to slip . . . or their old lady starts demanding new things, you know, like they always do. . . . They slow down on the route, maybe lose some customers. They'll buy a new car, boat, or motor home, and then mysteriously develop a bad back. But you know something's up when you find out that they just took out insurance on all their loans, insured to the teeth. . . . They freak out when they realize how much debt they're in. . . . They have two years of disability. It's funny, but there are a lot of guys who are miraculously healed at the end of those two years. You have to take them back, too, if they get a full-duty release.

This type of worker is usually married with no children. And he rarely owns his own home. A worker with a big mortgage and children tends not to entertain thoughts of malingering because his reduced salary would be insufficient to meet all his expenses. But the driver who spends considerable money on leisure-time possessions may perceive disability compensation as sufficient to cover the boat or camper payments, but also providing the free time to enjoy these possessions.

The second form of malingering begins with a real job-related injury that teaches the worker the benefits of compensation. He forestalls the rehabilitation process in order to enjoy the "free ride" offered by compensation (see also Sternbach, 1974: 60). Bill relates the history of one driver who followed such a pattern:

> Pedro was one of the hardest working guys I ever saw. He pulled his back, I guess, but didn't slow down like I told him to do. He just wouldn't take a few days off. . . . Well, look, he saw that he could make two-thirds of his wages and all that.

... For the first time in his life, he's got it easy [laugh], so you know he's not rushing back to work.

With either form of malingering, the worker perceives disability compensation as an easy way out of personal troubles.

OCCUPATIONAL MEDICINE AND CHRONIC PAIN

Disability compensation is rapidly becoming big business in the United States. There are currently 2.9 million Americans drawing disability benefits under Social Security alone. Total cost for all disability coverage is estimated to range from $20 to $30 billion (see Finneson, 1977: 37). As mentioned earlier, the chronic pain center concept has only come to fruition due to the availability of insurance carriers willing to pay for this service as part of their workmen's coverage.[3] As the American work ethic slips, many people are viewing this version of the welfare state as one way of beating the system. For this reason, it is virtually impossible to even estimate how many blue-collar manual laborers experience real job-related chronic pain.

Traditionally, occupational medicine has focused upon two facets of health care for the worker. One facet has been rehabilitation of injured or diseased workers; the other has been the elimination of environmental threats to the worker's health (e.g., eliminating industrial toxins and unsafe working conditions; see Hunter, 1969). The increasing cost of these programs, however, is forcing employers to concentrate their attention more on the individual worker's health before the advent of problems. Thus we witness a growth in *preventive* health care for workers. In terms of potential musculoskeletal/chronic pain problems, programs have been developed for preemployment screening of manual laborers to eliminate those workers most liable to back injuries (Chaffin et al., 1978) and for exercise strengthening (Everett, 1979).

Occupational medicine for the blue-collar manual laborer is beginning to resemble the preventive care offered the professional athlete. The preventive aspect of sports medicine is necessary because of the professional athlete's high value to his organization. Increased communication between the two forms of occupational medicine could greatly benefit the manual laborer. Sports medicine has been at the forefront of innovative treatments and therapies. It is clear, for example, that many manual laborers could greatly reduce the risk of back and leg injuries by engaging in some of the more sophisticated stretching exercises that are now routine in the professional athlete's pregame preparation. The point is that employers have to adapt to the fact that the terms "manual labor" and "cheap labor" can no longer be used interchangeably.

NOTES

1. Metaphor has been a fascinating topic of discussion among intellectuals for centuries. Even Plato and Aristotle attempted to denote its true nature. Positions have ranged from viewing all speech as metaphor (e.g., Nietzche) to viewing metaphor as a distinct element of language (e.g., Plato). Ricoeur (1977) provides the most comprehensive discussion of this topic.

2. I base my use of the term "subculture" on Fine and Kleinman's (1979) discussion. They define subculture as a set of understandings, behaviors, and artifacts used by particular groups and diffused through interlocking group networks. Identification with the values of the group, which is continually being revised through interaction, is the motivation for socialization into the subculture. There are two aspects of Fine and Kleinman's discussion that are crucial to understanding why I classify the blue-collar manual laborers' peer group as a subculture. First, identification with the group is variable across situations. The tavern clientele occupy many roles in addition to that one. Some manual laborers have less identification with the tavern milieu and more with the church or the family. My analysis is based on those workers who identify strongly with the tavern. Second, the authors note

how cultural transmission of subcultural values occurs through interpersonal communication, in lieu of media access. The central point of this chapter is that the manual laborers utilize the existing conversational format of the tavern to construct topics relevant to issues of health and illness.

3. Kotarba (1981) is an examination of the chronic pain center movement as an organizational response by disability compensation carriers and the Social Security Administration to the tremendous costs of job-related injury. Unlike other forms of social control, the pain center must induce its clients to comply with its program. Thus the injured worker simply believes that the center operates primarily to ease his or her suffering, when in fact its primary purpose is to return workers back to productivity.

7

PHYSICIANS, PATIENTS, AND PAIN:
AN OVERVIEW

In this study, I have surveyed the sociological aspects of the chronic pain experience. As an ongoing sensation of embodied discomfort that fails to respond to normal medical intervention, chronic pain is worthy of sociological analysis because the process of coping with it—in terms of seeking effective meaning for it and reconciling it with normal, everyday activities—is inherently social. A multiperspectival approach to the social meanings of chronic pain allows us to see how different audiences—including health care workers of various sorts, family members, coworkers, and employers, as well as the pain-afflicted person—attempt to make sense of this dilemma. Throughout this study, two distinct features of the chronic pain phenomenon keep recurring—*complexity* and *conflict.*

The enormous complexity of the chronic pain experience is readily seen in the way it affects virtually every aspect of the sufferer's life. In light of the fact that chronic pain rarely is life threatening and normally acts as a background or contextual element in one's daily life, this pervasiveness is of a different quality than that associated with catastrophic illness. Cancer or major cardiovascular disease, for example, can totally disrupt a person's social roles, especially when it requires long-term hospitalization (see Rosengren and Lefton, 1969). Occupational careers can be interrupted, status in the family can be undermined severely, and so forth. The person with chronic pain, on the other hand, ordinarily has the capability and motivation to maintain and meet normal social responsibilities, but must accommodate these demands with fairly constant physical discomfort. As we have seen, pain-afflicted people develop strategies for reconciling pain with sexual activities, work, family finances, self-esteem among peers, and so on.[1]

Complexity is also present in the enormous impact the chronic pain phenomenon has on all levels of the health care system. It has contributed to increasing disenchantment with organized medicine in our society, in terms of both its theoretical understanding of health and illness and its clinical effectiveness. Many paramedical workers have utilized the need for effective pain care as a vehicle for professional growth and to distance themselves from the physician's dominance. Complementary or alternative healers owe much of their success, if not their existence, to the pain care void. Finally, the high cost of pain care places a tremendous burden on insurance carriers and on the Social Security Administration, especially in regard to job-related disability claims for which the legal industry, not the patient, has become the primary beneficiary.

Although conflict can emerge between the pain-afflicted person and a range of significant others (e.g., spouse or employer) in the course of the coping process, conflict is most apparent in relationships with physicians. The genesis of this conflict lies in the disillusionment many pain-afflicted people have with the previously taken-for-granted powers of modern medicine. The outward manifestations of this conflict, at least on the part of the patient, are strategies to manipulate physicians, doctor hopping, and consideration of alternative health care options that include unorthodox and often discreditable modalities. It is clear, though, that this disillusionment cannot completely negate dependence on the physician due to medicine's cultural, scientific, and especially political preeminence in our society: The disillusioned patient may *need* physicians if only for their power to write prescriptions or to legally certify disability. What we do find is a shift in the nature or *essence* of the physician/patient relationship over the course of a lengthy pain career, particularly as this relationship is affected by changes in patient expectations.

In order to explore the theoretical significance of this shift, it would be useful to gauge the fit between the chronic pain experience and the sociological literature on the physician/patient relationship. In medical sociology, there are four major theoretical perspectives on this relationship: *functionalist, Marxist, interactionist,* and *decision-making* models.[2] Each model is derived from a more comprehensive paradigm or set of assumptions on the nature of social order and social life. Likewise, each model creates a metaphorical image of this relationship by accentuating one key aspect of physician/patient interaction. The strength of any metaphor, whether it be scientific or artistic, lies in its useful illumination of a phenomenon, as Brown (1977b) reminds us, and this criterion will be the basis for our discussion.

THE FUNCTIONALIST MODEL: PARSONS'S SICK ROLE

Parsons (1951) was the first sociologist to apply a distinctly sociological conceptualization to society's response to illness. In his efforts to formulate a comprehensive theory of society, Parsons was very much concerned with the mechanisms used to *integrate* all facets of society (i.e., how to keep society functioning well). Society is made up of a set of highly interdependent roles or positions in the social structure. A person naturally occupies several roles simultaneously (e.g., wife, mother, legal secretary, Baptist, and P.T.A. president), but the point is that any person is obliged to fulfill the expectations of each role occupied. Failure to live up to these expectations is considered "wrong" and, in sociological parlance, deviant behavior. Parsons argued that any society must control deviance in order to survive. In this respect, illness can be seen as a type of deviant behavior because it can preclude the fulfillment of normal role expectations. For example, a woman who becomes bedridden by illness can't fulfill her obligations as wife, mother, employee, and so on. The other family members may feel the strain of assuming her duties in addition to their own, thus threatening the integrity of the family as a social unit.

Society, therefore, must control illness by minimizing its pervasiveness and getting the sick back to normal as soon as possible. Modern Western societies are able to control illness by establishing a special social position that Parsons calls the *sick role* (1951: 436). There are four distinct expectations placed on a person who is considered to be legitimately ill and, thus, allowed to occupy the sick role. Two are rights afforded sick people by the groups to which they belong. Since legitimate illness is presumed to be beyond an individual's control, *the sick person is not held responsible for his or her condition.* Some sort of healing intervention is needed beyond the individual's personal motivation to get well. Moreover, *the sick person has the right to claim exemption from normal obligations and responsibilities.* Groups respond to a member's incapacitation either by allowing the fulfillment of less important duties to lapse or by providing alternative means for their execution, as is the case when an employer hires temporary help to "cover" for a sick employee.[3]

The temporary nature of the sick role is reflected in two obligations placed on the sick person. *The sick person is expected to try to get well as soon as possible.* Exemption from normal responsibilities is contingent on the desire to regain health, for the sick person should realize that illness is dysfunctional both personally and socially. In trying to get well, *the sick person is obliged to seek and cooperate with technically competent help.* Clearly, Parsons is referring here specifically to the physician and, generally, to the extensive medical system (e.g., hospitals, nurses, and pharmacists) organized around and controlled by the physician. The sick person is expected to place total responsibility for his or her illness in the hands of the physician, who is given license by society to determine "proper" health care (see also Parsons, 1975: 261-272).

Many writers who have tested Parsons's model empirically critique his formulation for not reflecting the great variation in actual patient responses to illness. For example, Gordon (1966) observed that minor illness tends to preclude the right to escape normal social obligations; Madsen (1973) observed that the cultural aspects of poverty preclude many poor people from placing total trust in physicians; and Kassebaum and Baumann (1965) observed that people with chronic conditions cannot be expected to try to get well. While this literature is impressive in its illustration of actual illness behavior, it does not adequately critique the intent of Parsons's model. Parsons's primary concern is *society's* response to illness, not the *individual's.* As Parsons argues, society's response to illness is both necessary and possible because its members share certain basic values and relate to each other in a spirit of cooperation. In regard to illness and disability, potential disruption of societal functioning is controlled because a majority of Americans are socialized into believing that organized medicine is the proper form of intervention during illness and that the physician, due to his or her professional stature and expertise, is the ultimate authority in caring for the sick. At this level of analysis, the variations in how people perceive and adapt to the sick role fade away, for most Americans ultimately do consult physicians for health care.

In a metaphorical sense, then, Parsons's concept of the sick role presents the image of a *paternalistic* relationship between the physician and patient. Just as society gives the parent authority over the child, it entrusts the physician with fiduciary power over the patient in what Parsons (1975: 266-267) views as a necessarily *asymetrical* way:

> This is to say in very general terms that the physician has been institutionally certified to be worthy of entrusting responsibility to in the field of the care of health. . . . I hasten to add that this fiduciary responsibility for the health of participants in the health care system . . . most definitely should be regarded as shared by sick persons. Indeed, the acceptance of the role of patient . . . may be said to impose a definite responsibility on the patient in working toward the common goals of the system as a whole.

The essence of the sick role concept, therefore, is the expectation of cooperation and trust by the patient in an inherently unequal relationship. The paternalistic metaphor is strongest when applied to the physician/patient relationship at the onset of pain. The typical pain patient assumes that the physician will be effective in eliminating the discomfort either because of the patient's previously successful encounters with medicine or because the patient has learned to expect medical success. The paternalistic metaphor weakens, however, as the pain persists and feelings of trust and cooperation are supplanted by distrust and anger. The situation is aggravated further when the physician begins to discredit the patient for either creating or enhancing the problem psychologically. The asymmetry of the relationship effectively breaks down to the degree that the patient gains independence by successfully developing strategies to manipulate the physician. Ironically, the fiduciary authority of the physician, which is supposedly intended to serve the interests of the patient, becomes a major impediment to open and constructive communication at that point in the chronic pain career when it is most needed.

It is also ironic to note how, on a societal level, the institution of medicine in fact hinders the productivity it is intended to protect. By acting in concert with the other segments of the disability compensation system (e.g., insurance carriers and lawyers), medicine actually *decreases* society's productivity by helping to produce a group of ex-workers who have little incentive to regain employment after a pain-related injury. Medicine contributes to this welfare state mentality by certifying disability in many instances when workers are either malingering or could be retrained for other types of work (see Chapter 6). Finally, we must consider the potential loss of productivity resulting from the notorious over-prescription of debilitating drugs and surgery, which are still medicine's primary response to chronic pain.[4]

THE MARXIST MODEL: MEDICINE AS BUSINESS

Medical sociologists of the Marxist (or critical) persuasion propose an alternative model for the societal-level analysis of medicine. Just as Parsons applied the idea of social role to illness management, critical writers apply Marxist notions of *capitalist exploitation* to this issue. Waitzkin (1971; and Waterman, 1974) has developed the most coherent Marxist model.[5] Waitzkin agrees with Parsons that the adoption of the sick role contributes to the stability of social institutions and the maintenance of social equilibrium. He disagrees with Parsons, however, on the desirability of the net effects of medicine as an institution of social control. Medicine serves the needs of the ruling class two ways, either by helping to "process" members of the suppressed classes (e.g., in military and industrial screening) or by diverting members of the suppressed classes away from a true understanding of the causes of their problems in life (e.g., in providing "sick leave" for teachers when their illness in fact is the result of the stress inherent in dealing with the repressive public school system).

While the Marxist analysis of the social control function of medicine is somewhat accurate if not unique to that perspective (see Zola, 1972), Marxist views on the economics of health care are more relevant to our discussion of the physician/patient relationship. Waitzkin (and Waterman, 1974: 86-89) argues that medicine in America is a monopoly that is, like other sectors of the capitalist economy, essentially *profit motivated* (see also Twaddle and Hessler, 1977: 39-40). Several problems arise when medicine's goal of making money overshadows its expected primary purpose of helping the sick. First, many poor people cannot afford decent health services (see also Kosa et al., 1969). Health care becomes a commodity instead of a right.[6] Second, medicine follows the imperialistic inclination of capitalism to forever expand both its influence in society and the market for its services. Hospitals, technology, overlap of services, and costs all proliferate as the medical empire expands. Third, medicine's definition of its domain has expanded until we now see its influence in virtually all areas of life, as exemplified by the requirement of medical certification for just about every possible status change (e.g., marriage, birth, employment). Marxists propose the elimination of the profit motive by either the socialization or nationalization of health care, so that all people can have access to as much health care as they think they need; health care would thus become a liberating experience.

In a metaphorical sense, then, the Marxist view of health care presents the image of an *economic* relationship between physician and patient. The patient/consumer desires a needed health service/commodity whose cost and availability are totally controlled by the physician/capitalist. The economic metaphor is weak when applied to the onset of pain, but becomes stronger as the chronic pain career evolves, at least in terms of the patient's perceived needs. At first, the economics of pain care is relatively unimportant for the typical patient. The initial cost of conservative treatment is relatively low, and in any event, is probably covered by personal/group health insurance or workmen's compensation. But as a series of expensive interventions such as surgeries, diagnostic tests, rehabilitation services, and drugs start to mount, the patient becomes increasingly aware of the cost-benefit ratio of pain care, especially when the insurance coverage nears the saturation point. Future surgery, for example, could be refused if the patient feels that its low probability of success does not justify its high economic—as well as emotional—cost. There is one limit, however, on the overall importance of the economic variable in the search for a cure. *In general, the pain-afflicted person will attempt virtually any treatment that appears likely to offer effective elimination of the pain, if at all economically feasible.* This is a major reason why acupuncture has become so popular, while treatment modalities such biofeedback, which are perceived as offering only pain control and are less expensive in general, are somewhat less popular.

The Marxist model is correct in noting that the relationship between physician and patient is more conflictful than cooperative, but the basis for this conflict among patients with chronic pain is more often effectiveness than cost. As a group, they have less perceived need for more and cheaper health care than for health care that works, thus calling into question the Marxist argument for an expansion of the health care system through socialization or nationalization.[7] Since the traditional services offered by medicine are largely ineffective in treating chronic pain, these patients need less medicine and more access to health care alternatives, in addition to increased control over decisions affecting their problems.

THE INTERACTIONIST MODEL:
THE SOCIAL CONSTRUCTION OF ILLNESS

The interactionist model of the physician/patient relationship is derived from the symbolic interactionist perspective on social life. In short, this perspective argues that social life is a fluid, symbolic reality that is created through the everyday interaction of people who attribute meaning to their world (see Adler and Adler, 1980). Accordingly, there are two types of reality associated with illness: biological and social. Medicine is concerned with the former by applying its own unique body of scientific knowledge to its amelioration. Sociology is concerned with the latter, for the diagnosis and treatment of disease are social acts based on socially constructed human knowledge that have consequences independent of their alleged biological bases. As Freidson (1970: 212), the major proponent of the interactionist perspective, puts it, illness is an *idea* and the sociological problem is the management "of the idea itself—how signs or symptoms get to be labeled or diagnosed as illness in the first place, how an individual gets to be labeled sick, and how social behavior is molded by the process of diagnosis and treatment."[8]

Like Parsons, Freidson sees the physician as an agent of social control, but one whose monopolistic power to create illness as an official social role is the product of success in political as well as scientific efforts. As an autonomous profession, medicine has complete control over its work, including relevant legal, ethical, scientific, and therapeutic issues. This authority not only determines the form of the entire medical world, but also heavily influences lay conceptions of health and illness.

The power of the physician to determine the use of medical labels such as "acute," "chronic," "health," and "illness," as well as who is allowed to occupy the sick role, is based upon the notion of *legitimacy* (Freidson, 1970: 237-240). Whereas Parsons assumes that all claims to the sick role are conditionally legitimate and contingent on the sick person's motivation to get well, Freidson contends that legitimacy becomes quite problematic for the chronically ill and the visibly handicapped. There are, in fact, three types of legitimacy controlled by physicians. *Conditional legitimacy,* as Parsons describes it, is imputed to the sick person who is expected to get well. The degree of exemption from normal responsibilities, though, depends on the relative seriousness of the illness, since a person is considered less incapacitated by a cold than by pneumonia. *Unconditional legitimacy* is imputed to the hopeless condition of the sick person not expected to get well. Again, the privileges afforded the patient on the seriousness of the condition and the degree of incapacitation. *Illegitimacy* is imputed to chronic conditions that negatively affect a person's identity. While people are not ordinarily held responsible for stigmatizing conditions such as stammering and epilepsy, they are nonetheless denied certain privileges because of their condition (e.g., access to certain occupations).

Friedson does not intend to imply that the social reality of illness is as static and as fixed as these analytical categories suggest. Normally, diseases have onsets, climaxes, outcomes, and continuously changing levels of seriousness. The process of becoming a sick person ordinarily follows a patterned sequence of illness definitions and interventions, or *career,* that is predominantly shaped by agents (i.e., physicians) and agencies (i.e., the medical system) provided by society to assist the sick person. During the process of making sense of embodied distress, the patient is relatively passive.[9]

In a metaphorical sense, then, the interactionist model according to Freidson presents the image of a *priestly* relationship between physician and patient. Like the Indian shaman who professes the magical power to expel evil spirits, the physician is empowered to create the idea of illness out of a complex array of amorphous symptoms or even no physical symptoms at all, as is often the case with mental illness. But Freidson fails to note that the physician's magic is much more powerful when applied to those disease states whose realities are more *symbolic* than *experiential.* Let's take an adult woman, for example, who consults her physician because she notices a small lump in her breast. The physician's diagnostic powers in this case are great and he can define the lump as malignant or benign. Since the subjective experience of the lump indicates neither, the woman is likely to agree with the physician's diagnosis because of both her socially acquired fear of cancer and her belief in the physician's expertise in these matters.

Chronic pain, on the other hand, is first and foremost a precognitive and visceral experience of bodily distress that the physician has less enforceable leeway in defining. In other words, the priestly metaphor is strongest when a *physiological* diagnosis is the focus of the physician/patient encounter. The typical pain patient accepts, for example, a diagnosis of "ruptured disc," since the experience of pain does not contradict the physician's expertise in this matter. The priestly metaphor is considerably weaker, however, when applied to an encounter dealing with *psychological* diagnosis, such as psychosomia, hypochondriasis, or depression. The embodied experience of pain contradicts a diagnosis that posits that the essence of pain emanates from the patient's psyche. Patients will ordinarily interpret a psychological diagnosis as doubting the veracity of their suffering and somehow blaming them for their problem. If the physician's diagnosis does not match the experience of the symptoms, it will be rejected and the search for adequate meaning will continue.[10]

THE DECISION-MAKING MODEL: THE RATIONAL PATIENT

The decision-making model, based on principles of social psychology, focuses on the process by which a patient eventually decides to consult a physician and conduct a therapeutic relationship. The key concept in this model is *illness behavior,* which Mechanic (1978) defines as "the way in which symptoms are perceived, evaluated, and acted upon by a person who recognizes some pain, discomfort, or other signs of organic malfunction." In developing a model of help seeking, Mechanic lists ten social-psychological variables that affect the response to illness, among the most crucial of which are: (1) "visibility, recognizability, or perceptual salience of deviant signs and symptoms"; (2) "the extent to which the symptoms are perceived as serious"; and (3) "availability of treatment resources, physical proximity, and psychological and monetary costs of taking action" (Mechanic, 1978: 268-269). Mechanic argues that the interplay of these ten variables explains why one person will ignore a condition while another person will allow the same condition to produce great social and psychological disability. Underlying Mechanic's model is the assumption that decisions made in response to these ten determinants are socially and culturally learned.

Suchman (1965b) expands Mechanic's decision-making model to account for the entire illness process. He lists five consecutive stages through which a person passes during the course of a discrete illness episode: (1) the symptom experience stage, (2) the assumption of the sick-role stage, (3) the medical care contact stage, (4) the dependent-patient role stage, and (5) recovery or rehabilitation stage. A sick person moves from one stage to the next as the result of a conscious decision to do so, in light of the perceived advantages of change. For example, a person decides to enter the dependent-patient stage when it appears rationally that the return to health is only possible if certain decision-making prerogatives are surrendered to the physician (Suchman, 1965b: 115).

In a metaphorical sense, then, the decision-making model presents the image of a *rationalist* relationship between physician and patient. The process of seeking health care is orderly, and patients react to symptoms in ways that are consistent with the attitudes and values of their social/cultural groups. This metaphor is probably strongest when applied to chronic pain patients' behavior at the onset of pain, but even at this point, patient discretion can be overridden if the pain originates with a traumatic and incapacitating injury and the patient is whisked off to a hospital emergency room. The decision-making model does not confront the central issue in chronic pain help seeking, which is not the initial decision to see a doctor, but the continuous search for medical and nonmedical help long after the initial consultation and intervention have failed. As we have seen, the search for a cure includes the perception and utilization of options that can be diametrically opposed to health care values learned through socialization.

Moreover, the image of the sick person as a calculated decision maker distorts the essence of the chronic pain experience, as well as any problematic illness experience. Most of our everyday activities are marked by fusions of feeling and thought, of the rational and the irrational (Johnson, 1975: 160-161; see also Douglas, 1977: 21-29). Our ability to decide rationally on courses of action is routinely undermined by the emotions, feelings, moods, and *semi*conscious thought evoked by the situation at hand. We should not assume that the sick person calmly weighs the costs and benefits of perceived options in situations permeated by agony, physical, and mental impairment, or even the fear of death or disability. They key to the rationalist bias of the decision-making model is the fact that it never considers the existential possibility of patient error in health care judgments. This model assumes that the ultimate correct decision is to consult a physician, but as we have seen, medical intervention can prolong if not worsen the experience of pain. In any event, the rational variables Mechanic and others discuss diminish in usefulness over the course of a lengthy chronic pain career as many patients come to be increasingly guided by a *blind hope* for a cure (Kotarba, 1975: 154-160) and good guesswork and chance taking.

Although pure rationality is less relevant than Mechanic and others would argue to the ongoing search for help, the *semblance* of rationality is very important to the pain-afflicted person's display of competence. To give others the impression that one deals with health problems haphazardly is to risk their moral discrediting (i.e., shaming), since our culture values highly thoughtful concern over matters of health and illness. This fact helps to explain why pain-afflicted people are so well versed in the professional and popular literature on pain control. Intellectual sophistication helps one rationally to "account for" (Lyman and Scott, 1970) what is in fact a very irrational decision.[11]

AN EXISTENTIAL MODEL OF THE
CHRONIC PAIN EXPERIENCE

The four sociological models we have analyzed, although contributing much to our overall understanding of the physician/patient relationship, provide incomplete if not distorted portraits of this relationship in regard to the chronic pain experience. The *essence* of this particular relationship lies not in any single, categorical dimension, but is found in the way each dimension waxes and wanes in importance over the course of a lengthy and uncertain condition. There are two reasons why these models fail to account for this fluidity.

First, these models are based largely on the writers' understanding of physicians' input into the relationship, in terms of either physicians' own behavior and/or their perceptions of how patients do or should behave. Regardless of whether this input is seen as producing a paternalistic, economic, priestly, or rationalist relationship, it is assumed that this input is fairly stable and consistent over time, due to the professional, and therefore predictable, nature of the physician's role in our society.[12] The present study indicates, though, that changes in the overall conduct of the relationship—including engagement, withdrawal, and the emergence of conflict—are closely related to, and reflect, changes in the *patients'* definitions of what their doctors have to offer.

Second, and more important, these models do not reflect the true *existential* nature of the chronic pain experience. As existential social thought reminds us, everyday social life and efforts to create social order consist of the uncertain, emergent, often conflictful, and always difficult search for meaning in an intrinsically meaningless world. Social meanings are problematic because the context within which any social event occurs is of fundamental importance in determining the meaning of that event (Douglas, 1970: 35-44; Kotarba, 1979). Similarly, chronic pain patients, whose essential purpose (like all patients) for encountering physicians is to obtain meaning for their condition, will define each encounter according to the practical (i.e., contextual) considerations at hand. We have already seen how patients' definitions shift gradually over the course of their pain careers, but these definitions can also vary immediately and situationally. This is especially true for those patients who consult several healers concurrently for different kinds of health care meanings, so that we can expand our discussion to include nonmedical as well as medical healers. For example, the following is a plausible, composite scenario.

A middle-aged man with chronic low-back pain very passively consults his family physician once a month in order to obtain prescriptions for analgesic drugs and to receive authoritative confirmation of his condition for the doubters in his family (paternalistic considerations). When the physician alludes to the possibility that the man may be compounding his problem by failing to adjust emotionally to his pain, the man retreats to the solace of is minister, who tells him that his pain is a gift from God that will ensure happiness in the afterlife (priestly considerations). Once a week, the man consults a chiropractor who not only provides an audience to which the man can vent his anger toward the physician, but whose manipulations are less expensive as well as less terrifying than the back surgery the physician has been suggesting (economic considerations). Finally, on the day before he is scheduled for a routine company physical examination, the man will discuss strategies with his wife—or his friends in the bar—for concealing his condition from the company physician in order to minimize risk to his upcoming promotion (rationalist considerations).

Thus far, we have seen how changes in the nature of the physician/patient relationship relate to changes in the patients' definition of the purpose and potential of the relationship. There is a third element in this process that helps explain how patients acquire the *idea* that they can in fact gain autonomy and discretion in dealing with and defining healers. I am referring to the reconstruction of self that occurs during the chronic pain experience. Strauss and Glaser (1975: 52-53) have shown how people with various kinds of chronic illness often experience unstable social arrangements, brought about by a developing yet uncertain disease trajectory. Consequently, the chronically ill person's views of him- or herself cannot remain unaltered. The sense of self can become hopelessly unmoored and negative, especially if the disease or its symptoms are morally stigmatized by others. In the present study, we have seen how the pain-afflicted person's self-conception can be damaged, especially in terms of the loss of self-esteem experienced when the pain threatens the competent fulfillment of social roles, or when a physician stigmatizes the patient with a diagnosis of psychological disturbance.

Over the course of a chronic pain career, the individual attempts to nullify negative connotations of self by shifting the loci of self from what Turner (1976) refers to as *institutions* to *impulse*. To paraphrase Turner's insightful discussion, we could say that the person whose self-conception is rooted in institutions finds satisfaction and reward in following established social rules and values. Loyalty to group obligations and rational control over one's behavior are the essence of self-worth. The person whose self-conception is rooted in impulse finds satisfaction through rejection of social rules and established values, which are perceived as deceptive and constraining. The "true" self is something to be discovered, the result of spontaneous desires and behavior. If we apply Turner's model to the chronic pain experience, we can see how the shift in locus of self affects the definition of relationships with healers. At the onset of pain, the individual attempts to protect the self by being institutions oriented, that is, by grounding the self in the social role of the "good" patient. As Turner (1976: 1005) states, "The discovery of self through immersion in an institutional framework makes the world predictable and the rich body of objects opens up a new world of gratifications." But as the pain persists, the patient may begin to feel betrayed and begin withdrawal of personal investment in the "proper" course of action. At this point, the self is uncertain and unable to find security in the traditional definition of the good patient. The self then is necessarily freed to adhere to psychic, mystical, folk, or even irrational conceptions that reflect optional healing experiences. It is also freed to adhere to an *instrumental* conception that allows it to find comfort and possible reward in the manipulation of healing relationships. Previous belief in the traditional physician/patient relationship as *being* the correct one evolves into a much more impulsive belief that the next healing relationship *may be* the right one.

Turner designed his model to explain the historic shift in self-conception occurring within our society over the past several decades.[13] My application of his model to the chronic pain experience is a microcosmic illustration of this process of change as it occurs during the course of an individual's pain career. But there is yet another quality of self, even more basic than the cognitive dimension of self-conception, that underlies the entire coping process—*embodiment.* As existential social thought reminds us, corporality is the overwhelming fact of human existence (Merleau-Ponty: 1962; see also Kotarba, 1979: 357). Being-within-the-world means that feelings and our immediate perceptions of reality precede rational thought and symbol use, and in fact, activate them. The experience of embodiment is the center of our universe, the criterion by which all social meanings are eventually gauged.

Likewise, the primordial perception of pain not only activates the search for meaning, but also serves as the criterion by which available meanings are interpreted. Adequate health care meanings must lead to control of the physical discomfort as well as a reduction in the threat posed by pain to one's bodily integrity, the source of our being. Adequate lay meanings must help the individual cope with pain in everyday life and restore harmony between body and world. In either case, the *active* self will override inadequate meanings, regardless of the social, medical, or moral authority enforcing them, and seek a more useful understanding of the dilemma elsewhere.

A PROSPECTIVE LOOK AT THE CHRONIC PAIN PHENOMENON

I would like to conclude this study on an optimistic—and I hope, realistic—note. I firmly believe that the future bodes well for the chronic pain phenomenon. Several developments in the field of pain care should help alleviate the widespread suffering caused by this affliction.

Research on new modes of pain control is most promising, especially that being conducted on *endorphins*. Endorphins are natural chemicals, or peptides, found in the brain. Researchers have identified five major endorphins that seem to mimic the analgesic effects of morphine. It has been suggested that acupuncture may be effective in reducing pain because it releases endorphins into the system (Cheng and Pomeranz, 1979). Much of the excitement emanating from this research lies in its promise of utilizing the body's own natural healing powers, an approach to pain care that can eliminate the harmful side effects of chemical and surgical interventions.

Acupuncture and chiropractic are gaining legal if not medical legitimacy. More and more states are approving the independent practice of acupuncture, as exemplified by a recent (1980) court ruling in Texas that is bringing previously indigenous practitioners of this art into the open health care marketplace. Chiropractic's efficacy in treating specific kinds of chronic pain, such as that related to the sacral region, may be a factor in reducing tension between medicine and chiropractic. Indeed, one scholarly observer of the chiropractic profession argues that it may eventually evolve into a limited medical practice much like dentistry and podiatry (Wardwell, 1978). Finally, there are indications that the chronic pain center movement is retracting from its earlier unviable commitment to behavior modification and expanding its range of services to include more humanistic modalities. A benefit of this change would be to open pain centers to a broader range of pain patients, as opposed to many centers' current policy of limiting themselves to disability compensation cases that are overrepresented by psychological disorders for which behavioral strategies are best suited.

Even with the good prospects for progress in the field of pain care, I would still expect the theoretical findings of this study to be relevant. The movement toward professionalization among paramedical workers involved with pain care will continue (although at a fairly slow pace due to the entrenched power of organized medicine) as their identities within the health care system become more formalized. The health care marketplace should continue to expand as complementary options to medicine proliferate and their perceived usefulness to patients widens. But in light of the fact that the overall prospect for eliminating pain and disease in our lives is dim, the search for health care meanings—in all its conflictful, secretive, strategic, and hopeful dimensions—will continue.

NOTES

1. Strauss and Glaser (1975: 58-65) discuss this accommodation in terms of "normalizing." Although their discussion deals with a range of chronic illnesses, their analysis can be applied usefully to chronic pain. Strategies for normalizing include distracting the attention of others away from the symptoms, convincing others that one can still function normally in spite of the condition, and convincing others that one's assessment of the condition is legitimate.

2. There are several other sociological models of the physician/patient relationship that, although theoretically significant, have had less impact on medical sociology and, therefore, will not be considered in our discussion (see, for example, Szasz and Hollender, 1956, and Hayes-Bautista, 1976).

3. The large pools of substitute teachers maintained by public school districts provide the clearest examples of the institutionalization of temporary help.

4. Siegler and Osmond (1973) present one of the most insightful as well as literary discussions of the sick role, borrowing illustrations from the medical sociology literature and Thomas Mann's *The Magic Mountain.* The authors contend that there are in fact eight different social roles available to or imposed on the ill person.

5. Conrad and Kern (1981) is a comprehensive collection of essays on health and illness from the Marxist or critical perspective.

6. It is clear, though, that the long-term trend is toward equalization of physician's services use rate among all socioeconomic class groupings, thanks to programs like Medicare and Medicaid (Monteiro, 1973). The resultant economic issue, according to Carlson (1975: 40), is the increased economic burden of supporting this quasi-socialized health care system felt by the middle and working classes.

7. Cooper (1975) and Illich (1976) discuss the problems inherent in the over-medicalization of our society.

8. Freidson based his model on the labeling theory of deviance. In short, this theory proposes that deviance is not a quality inherent in any social act or condition, as Parsons assumes regarding illness, but is the application of potentially discrediting definitions that are created by various social groups and enforced by agents of social control (see Kotarba, 1980a).

9. Lorber (1972) modifies Freidson's model to account for the power occasionally utilized by patients in contending with physicians. This power comes about in the negotiation of illness reality. For example, a person may define him- or herself as healthy, yet construct a performance of illness for a doctor in order to achieve the sick role (i.e., malingering). On the other hand, a person who is self-defined as ill may present him- or herself to the physician as healthy in order to continue leading as normal a life as possible.

10. There have been many empirical applications of Freidson's ideas and the symbolic interactionist perspective to the study of illness, the most interesting of which is the work of Strauss and Glaser (1975) and their students. Strauss and Glaser develop the concept of career, or trajectory as they call it, to account for the course of an illness as defined by all participants to it, not only the physician. Fagerhaugh and Strauss (1977) discuss how the institutionalization of the medical label "acute illness" creates problems in the hospital management of pain.

11. According to Lyman and Scott (1970), an account is a linguistic element employed whenever an action is subject to questioning by others. Specifically, a "justification" account is one that asserts the positive value of an act in face of a possible claim to the contrary. The pain-afflicted person may use his or her knowledge of healing to convince others that a seemingly irrational search for meaning is in fact based on more than a simple hunch or hope. Rosenstock (1960) provides an early version of the decision-making model that greatly influenced the work of Mechanic and Suchman. Fabrega (1973) expands Suchman's model to include nine stages of illness behavior. Operating through an anthropological framework,

he eliminates consideration of sociocultural variables in order to make his model applicable to any number of cultures.

12. The degree to which physicians modify their perceptions of relationships with long-term patients is a much neglected topic of study in medical sociology, but beyond the scope of the present study. Stewart and Buck's (1977) analysis of the development of the practitioners knowledge of the patient's problems is a rare exception.

13. There are, of course, other sociological analyses of recent trends in the process of self-construction. Douglas (1977: 3-73) argues that modern history is marked by a revolt of brute being. Brute being is the core of an individual's innermost feelings and perceptions. Furthermore,

> Modern man is rediscovering his brute being, freeing his being, and thereby willing and creating a new self and a new world. . . . Everywhere modern men have asserted their human existence over other-worldly essences, their subjective beings over the absolutist domination of external objects, their creative feelings over repressive moralism . . . their self-willed desires over externally imposed repressions.

Zurcher (1977) has identified the *mutable self* as a phenomenon unique to the present generation. The mutable self refers to the contemporary person's need to be ready and able to quickly shift self-conceptions as rapid social change occurs and traditional self-conceptions become constraints to adaptation.

References

Adler, Peter and Patricia A. Adler
1980   "Symbolic Interactionism." Pp. 20-61 in Jack D. Douglas et al. Introduction to the Sociologies of Everyday Life. Boston: Allyn & Bacon.

Allen, Gillian and Roy Wallis
1976   "Pentacostalists As a Medical Minority." Pp. 110-137 in Roy Wallis and Peter Morley (Eds.) Marginal Medicine. New York: Macmillan.

Altheide, David L. and John M. Johnson
1979   Modern Bureaucratic Propaganda. Boston: Allyn & Bacon.
1977   "Counting Souls: A Study of Counseling At Evangelical Crusades." Pacific Sociological Review 20: 323-348.

American Medical Association
1969   "Chiropractic Condemned." Journal of the American Medical Association 208: 352.

Aquinas, Thomas
1964   Summa Theologiae. Blackfriars (trans.). New York: McGraw-Hill.

Balint, Michael
1957   The Doctor, His Patient and the Illness. London: Pitman.

Ball, Donald and John W. Loy (Eds.)
1975   Sport and Social Order. Reading, MA: Addison-Wesley.

Bandura, A.
1974   "Behavior Theories and Models of Man." American Psychologist 29: 859-869.

Bauman, Edward
1979   The Holistic Health Handbook. Berkeley, CA: And/Or Press.

Beecher, Henry K.
1959   Measurement of Subjective Responses. New York: Oxford University Press.

Bellah, Robert N.
1976   "New Religious Consciousness and the Crisis in Modernity." Pp. 333-352 in Charles Y. Glock and Robert N. Bellah (Eds.) The New Religious Consciousness. Berkeley: University of California Press.

Berkman, Barbara
1977   "Innovations for Social Services in Health Care." Pp. 92-126 in Francine Sobey (Ed.) Changing Roles in Social Work Practice. Philadelphia: Temple University Press.

Berne, Eric
 1964   Games People Play. New York: Grove.
Bliss, Ann A. and Eva D. Cohen (Eds.)
 1977   The New Health Professionals. Germantown, MD: Aspen.
Blumer, H.
 1969   Symbolic Interactionism. Englewood Cliffs, NJ: Prentice-Hall.
Bonica, John J.
 1974   "Therapeutic Acupuncture and Implications for American Medicine."
         Journal of the American Medical Association 228: 18-27.
 1953   The Management of Pain. Philadelphia: Lea & Febiger.
Bracht, Neil F. (Ed.)
 1978   Social Work in Health Care: A Guide to Professional Practice. New York:
         Haworth.
Brimble, Phillip
 1979   "Nature Has Its Own 'Painkiller.'" The Kansas City Times, Missouri (Feb-
         ruary 22): 0-1.
Brown, Carol A.
 1975   "Women Workers in the Health Service Industry." International Journal of
         Health Services 5: 173-184.
Brown, Richard
 1977a   "The Emergence of Existential Thought." Pp. 77-100 in Jack D. Douglas
         and John M. Johnson (Eds.) Existential Sociology. New York: Cambridge
         University Press.
 1977b   A Poetic for Sociology. New York: Cambridge University Press.
Bullough, Vern and Bonnie Bullough
 1965   The Emergence of Modern Nursing. London: Macmillan.
Burns, Eveline M.
 1973   "Health Services for Tomorrow: Trends and Issues." American Behavioral
         Scientist 15: 713-721.
Butcher, James N. (Ed.)
 1969   MMPI: Research Development and Clinical Applications. New York:
         McGraw-Hill.
Cannon, J. Timothy, John C. Liebeskind, and Hanan Frenk
 1978   "Neural and Neuro-Chemical Mechanisms of Pain Inhibition." Pp. 27-47 in
         R. Sternbach (Ed.) The Psychology of Pain. New York: Raven.
Carlson, Rick J.
 1975   The End of Medicine. New York: John Wiley.
Casey, Kenneth L.
 1973   "Pain: A Current View of Neural Mechanisms." American Scientist 61:
         194-200.
Cavan, Sherri
 1966   Liquor License: An Ethnography of Bar Behavior. Chicago: Aldine.
Chaffin, Don B., Gary D. Herrin, and W. Monroe Keyserling
 1978   "Preemployment Strength Testing." Journal of Occupational Medicine 20:
         403-408.

Chapman, C. Richard, Anders E. Sola, and John J. Bonica
1979   "Illness Behavior and Depression Compared in Pain Center and Private Practice Patients." Pain 6: 1-7.

Cheng, R. and B. Pomeranz
1979   "Electroacupuncture Analgesia Could Be Mediated by at Least Two Pain Relieving Mechanisms: Endorphin and Non-Endorphin Systems." Life Sciences 25: 1957-1962.

Cicourel, Aaron V.
1974   Cognitive Sociology. New York: Macmillan.
1964   Method and Measurement. New York: Macmillan.

Cleland, Virginia
1976   "Developing a Doctoral Program." Nursing Outlook 24: 631-635.

Cobb, Beatrice
1958   "Why Do People Detour to Quacks?" Pp. 283-87 in E. Gartley Jaco (Ed.) Patients, Physicians, and Illness. New York: Macmillan.

Cockerham, William C.
1978   Medical Sociology. Englewood Cliffs, NJ: Prentice-Hall.

Coe, Rodney
1978   Sociology of Medicine. New York: McGraw-Hill.

Combs, Arthur, et al.
1971   Helping Relationships: Basic Concepts for the Helping Professions. Boston: Allyn & Bacon.

Conrad, Peter and Rochelle Kern (Eds.)
1981   The Sociology of Health and Illness: Critical Perspectives. New York: St. Martin's.

Cooper, Michael H.
1975   Rationing Health Care. London: Halsted.

Cosa, John, Aaron Antonovsky, and Irving K. Zola (Eds.)
1969   Poverty and Health. Cambridge, MA: Harvard University Press.

Costa, E. and M. Trabucchi (Eds.)
1978   The Endorphins. New York: Raven.

Cousins, Norman
1979   Anatomy of an Illness. New York: W. W. Norton.

Cowie, James B. and Julian Roebuck
1975   An Ethnography of a Chiropractic Clinic. New York: Macmillan.

Crowley, Dorothy M.
1962   Pain and Its Alleviation. Los Angeles: UCLA School of Nursing.

Davidson, Park O. (Ed.)
1976   The Behavioral Management of Anxiety, Depression and Pain. New York: Brunner/Mazel.

Davis, Fred
1972   Illness, Interaction, and the Self. Belmont, CA: Wadsworth.
1966   The Nursing Profession. New York: John Wiley.
1963   Passage Through Crisis: Polio Victims and Their Families. Indianapolis: Bobbs-Merrill.

1961   "Deviance Avowal: The Management of Strained Interaction by the Visibly Handicapped." Social Problems 9: 120-132.

Davis, Fred and Virginia L. Olesen
1965   "The Career Outlook of Professionally Educated Women: The Case of Collegiate Student Nurses." Psychiatry 28: 334-345.

Denton, John A.
1978   Medical Sociology. Boston: Houghton Mifflin.

Descartes, Rene
1955   The Philosophical Works of Descartes. (Trans. Elizabeth S. Haldane and G.R.T. Ross) New York: Dover.

Dimond, E. Grey
1971   "More Than Herbs and Acupuncture." Saturday Review (September 18): 17-19.

Dintenfass, Julius
1973   "The Administration of Chiropractic in the New York City Medicaid Program." Medical Care 11: 47-48.

Dorken, Herbert (Ed.)
1976   The Professional Psychologist Today. San Francisco: Jossey-Bass.

Dorken, Herbert and J. Frank Whiting
1974   "Psychologists as Health-Service Providers." Professional Psychology 5: 309-319.

Douglas, Jack D.
1977   "Existential Sociology" Pp. 3-73 in Jack D. Douglas and John M. Johnson (Eds.) Existential Sociology. New York: Cambridge University Press.
1976   Investigative Social Research. Beverly Hills, CA: Sage.
1971   American Social Order. New York: Macmillan.
1970   Understanding Everyday Life. Chicago: Aldine.
1967   The Social Meanings of Suicide. Princeton, NJ: Princeton University Press.

Douglas, Jack D., Patricia A. Adler, Peter Adler, Andrea Fontana,
        C. Robert Freeman, and Joseph A. Kotarba
1980   Introduction to the Sociologies of Everyday Life. Boston: Allyn & Bacon.

Douglas, Jack D. and John M. Johnson (Eds.)
1977   Existential Sociology. New York: Cambridge University Press.

Dubos, René
1969   Man, Medicine, and Environment. New York: Mentor.
1959   The Mirage of Health: Utopian Progress and Biological Change. New York: Doubleday.

Edwards, Harry
1973   Sociology of Sport. Homewood, IL: Dorsey.

Encyclopedia of Sports and Sciences and Medicine
1971   New York: American College of Sports Medicine.

Everett, Michael D.
1979   "Strategies for Increasing Employees' Level of Exercise and Physical Fitness." Journal of Occupational Medicine 21: 463-467.

Fabrega, Horacio, Jr.
1973   "Toward a Model of Illness Behavior." Medical Care 6: 470-484.

Fagerhaugh, Shizuko Y. and Anselm Strauss
  1977 Politics of Pain Management. Reading, MA: Addison-Wesley.
Feinstein, B., J. C. Luce, and J.N.K. Langton
  1954 "The Influence of Phantom Limbs." Pp. 216-239 in P. Klopsteg and P. Wilson (Eds.) Human Limbs and Their Substitutes. New York: McGraw Hill.
Field, Mark George
  1957 Doctor and Patient in Soviet Russia. Cambridge, MA: Harvard University Press.
Fine, Gary A. and Sheryl Kleinman
  1979 "Subculture: An Interactionist Analysis." American Journal of Sociology 85: 1-20.
Fink, Arthur E. (Ed.)
  1974 The Field of Social Work. New York: Holt, Rinehart & Winston.
Finneson, Bernard E.
  1977 "Clinical Portrait of a Patient with Industry-Related Chronic Low Back Pain." Pp. 37-43 in Pierre L. LeRoy (Ed.) Current Concepts in Management of Chronic Pain. New York: Symposia Specialists.
Fisk, James W.
  1977 The Painful Neck and Back. Springfield, IL: Charles C Thomas.
Fordyce, Wilbert E.
  1976 Behavioral Methods for Chronic Pain and Illness. St. Louis: Mosby.
Freeman, Howard E., Sol Levine, and Leo G. Reeder (Eds.)
  1972 Handbook of Medical Sociology. Englewood Cliffs, NJ: Prentice-Hall.
Freese, Arthur S.
  1974 "Pain Clinic." Physician's World (July): 29-31.
Freidson, Eliot
  1970 Profession of Medicine. New York: Dodd, Mead.
  1966 "Disability as Social Deviance." Pp. 71-99 in Marvin B. Sussman (Ed.) Sociology and Rehabilitation. Washington, DC: American Sociological Association.
Garfield, Sol L.
  1974 Clinical Psychology. Chicago: Aldine.
  1965 "Historical Introduction." Pp. 125-140 in B. B. Wolman (Ed.) Handbook of Clinical Psychology, New York: McGraw-Hill.
Germain, Carel B.
  1973 "An Ecological Perspective in Casework Practice." Social Casework 54: 323-330.
Goffman, Erving
  1963 Stigma. Englewood Cliffs, NJ: Prentice-Hall.
  1959 The Presentation of Self in Everyday Life. Garden City, NY: Doubleday.
Gold, Margaret
  1977 "A Crisis of Identity: The Case of Medical Sociology." Journal of Health and Social Behavior 18: 160-168.
Goode, William J.
  1960 "Encroachment, Charlatanism, and the Emerging Professions: Psychology, Sociology and Medicine." American Sociological Review 25: 902-914.

Gordon, Chad and Kenneth J. Gergen (Eds.)
1968   The Self in Social Interaction. New York: John Wiley.
Gordon, Gerald
1966   Role Theory and Illness. New Haven, CT: College and University Press.
Graham, Saxon
1974   "The Sociological Approach to Epidemiology." American Journal of Public Health 64: 1046-1049.
Gregory, Paul M.
1956   The Baseball Player: An Economic Study. Washington, DC: Public Affairs Press.
Guiora, Alexander Z. and Marvin A. Brandwin (Eds.)
1968   Perspectives in Clinical Psychology. Princeton, NJ: Van Nostrand.
Hadden, Stuart C. and Marilyn Lester
1980   "Ethnomethodology and Grounded Theory Methodology: An Integration of Topic and Method. Urban Life 9, 1: 3-33.
Haney, C. Allen and Anthony C. Colson
1980   "Ethical Responsibility in Physician-Patient Communication." Ethics in Science and Medicine 7: 27-36.
Hayes-Bautista, David E.
1976   "Termination of the Patient-Practitioner Relationship." Journal of Health and Social Behavior 17: 12-21.
Hilgard, Ernest R.
1978   "Hypnosis and Pain." Pp. 219-240 in Richard A. Sternbach (Ed.) The Psychology of Pain. New York: Raven.
Hilgard, Ernest R. and Josephine R. Hilgard
1975   Hypnosis in the Relief of Pain. Los Altos, CA: Kaufmann.
Hill, H. E., C. H. Kornetsky, H. G. Flanary, and A. Wilder
1952   "Effects of Anxiety and Morphine on the Discrimination of Intensities of Pain." Journal of Clinical Investigations 31: 473-480.
Houston, John P.
1976   Fundamentals of Learning. New York: Academic.
Hudson, James
1970   "Social Policy and Theoretical Sociology." Paper Presented at the Annual Meeting of the Mid-West Sociological Society, St. Louis.
Huizinga, John
1950   Homo Ludens: A Study of the Play Element in Culture. Boston: Beacon.
Hunter, D.
1969   The Diseases of Occupation. London: English Universities Press.
Hutchin, Kenneth C.
1965   Slipped Discs. New York: ARC Books.
Illich, Ivan
1976   Medical Nemesis. New York: Random House.
Irwin, John
1977   Scenes. Beverly Hills, CA: Sage.
Jaco, E. Gartly (Ed.)
1958   Patients, Physicians and Illness. New York: Macmillan.

Jakobivitz, Immanuel
1967   Jewish Medical Ethics. New York: Bloch.
Jacobs, Durand F.
1976   "Standards for Psychologists." Pp. 19-32 in Herbert Dorken (Ed.) The Professional Psychologist Today. San Francisco: Jossey-Bass.
Johnson, John M.
1975   Doing Field Research. New York: Macmillan.
Johnstone, Ronald L.
1975   Religion and Society in Interaction. Englewood Cliffs, NJ: Prentice-Hall.
Karlins, Marvin and Lewis M. Andrews
1972   Biofeedback. New York: Warner Books.
Kassebaum, Gene G. and Barbara O. Baumann
1965   "Dimensions of the Sick Role in Chronic Illness." Journal of Health and Human Behavior 6: 16-27.
Kelly, E. Lowell
1966   "Clinical Psychology: The Postwar Decade." Pp. 104-21 in I. N. Mensh (Ed.) Clinical Psychology: Science and Profession. New York: Macmillan.
Kemper, Theodore D.
1978   A Social Interactional Theory of Emotions. New York: John Wiley.
Koos, Earl L.
1954   The Health of Regionville. New York: Columbia University Press.
Kotarba, Joseph A.
1982   "One More for the Road: The Subversion of Labeling within the Tavern Subculture." In Jack D. Douglas (Ed.) Observations of Deviance. New York: Random House.
1981   "Chronic Pain Center: A Study of Voluntary Client Compliance and Entrepreneurship." American Behavioral Scientist 24: 786-800.
1980a   "Labeling Theory and Everyday Deviance." Pp. 82-112 in Jack D. Douglas et al. Introduction to the Sociologies of Everyday Life. Boston: Allyn & Bacon.
1980b   "Discovering Amorphous Social Experience: The Case of Chronic Pain." Pp. 57-67 in William B. Shaffir, Robert A. Stebbins, and Allan Turowetz (Eds.) Fieldwork Experience: Qualitative Approaches to Social Research. New York: St. Martin's.
1979   "Existential Sociology." Pp. 348-368 in Scott G. McNall (Ed.) Theoretical Perspectives in Sociology. New York: St. Martin's.
1977   "The Chronic Pain Experience." Pp. 257-272 in Jack D. Douglas and John M. Johnson (Eds.) Existential Sociology. New York: Cambridge University Press.
1975   "American Acupuncturists: The New Entrepreneurs of Hope." Urban Life 4: 149-177.
Kraus, Hans
1970   Clinical Treatment of Back and Neck Pain. New York: McGraw-Hill.
Kuby, Alma
1965   "The Chiropractic Patient." Unpublished Masters Paper. University of Chicago.

Kuhn, Thomas S.
1970   The Structure of Scientific Revolutions. Chicago: University of Chicago Press.

Landy, David (Ed.)
1977   Culture, Disease, and Healing. New York: Macmillan.

Leake, Chauncey D. and Milton Silverman
1966   Alcoholic Beverages in Clinical Medicine. Chicago: Year Book Medical Publishers.

Leavitt, Judith W. and Ronald L. Numbers (Eds.)
1978   Sickness and Health in America. Madison: University of Wisconsin Press.

LeMasters, E. E.
1975   Blue-Collar Aristocrats. Madison: University of Wisconsin Press.

Lenburg, Carrie B. (Ed.)
1975   Open Learning and Career Mobility in Nursing. St. Louis: Mosby.

Lennard, Henry L., Leon J. Epstein, Arnold Bernstein, and Donald C. Ransom
1971   Mystification and Drug Misuse. New York: Harper & Row.

LeRoy, Pierre L. (Ed.)
1977   Current Concepts in the Management of Chronic Pain. New York: Symposia Specialists.

LeShan, Lawrence
1964   "The World of the Patient in Severe Pain of Long Duration." Journal of Chronic Diseases 17: 119-126.

Lewis, C. S.
1961   The Problem of Pain. New York: Macmillan.

Lipowski, Z. J.
1970   "Physical Illness, The Individual and the Coping Process." Psychiatry and Medicine 1: 91-101.

Lorber, Judith
1972   "Deviance as Performance: The Case of Illness." Pp. 414-424 in Eliot Freidson and Judith Lorber (Eds.) Medical Men and Their Work. Chicago: Aldine.

Lovejoy, Arthur O.
1961   The Reason, The Understanding, and Time. Baltimore: Johns Hopkins University Press.

Lyman, S. and M. B. Scott
1970   A Sociology of the Absurd. Santa Monica, CA: Goodyear.

MacAndrew, Craig and R. B. Edgerton
1969   Drunken Comportment: A Social Explanation. Chicago: Aldine.

Madsen, William
1973   The Mexican-Americans of South Texas. New York: McGraw-Hill.

Maher, Charles
1978   "Playing with Pain: Medical Abuse or a Badge of Courage?" The Los Angeles Times (August 29): J1-J7.

Mandell, Arnold J.
1976   The Nightmare Season. New York: Random House.

Mann, Felix
1973   Acupuncture: The Ancient Chinese Art of Healing. New York: Random House.

Manning, Peter K. and Horatio Fabrega, Jr.
1973   "The Experience of Self and Body." Pp. 251-300 in George Psathas (Ed.)
        Phenomenological Sociology. New York: John Wiley.
Marcel, Gabriel
1952   Metaphysical Journal. (Trans. Bernard Wall.) Chicago: Regnery.
1951   The Mystery of Being. (Trans. Rene Hague.) Chicago: Regnery.
Mauksch, Hans O.
1972   "Nursing: Churning for a Change?" Pp. in Howard E. Freeman, et al. (Eds.)
        Handbook of Medical Sociology. Englewood Cliffs, NJ: Prentice-Hall.
McCaffery, Margo
1972   Nursing Management of the Patient With Pain. Philadelphia: Lippincott.
McCorkle, Thomas
1961   "Chiropractic: A Deviant Theory of Disease and Treatment." Human Or-
        ganization 20: 20-23.
McKeown, Thomas
1965   Medicine in Modern Society. London: Allen & Unwin.
Mechanic, David
1978   Medical Sociology. New York: Macmillan.
Mehan, Hugh and Houston Wood
1975   The Reality of Ethnomethodology. New York: John Wiley.
Meichenbaum, Donald and Dennis Turk
1976   "The Cognitive-Behavioral Management of Anxiety, Anger, and Pain."
        Pp. 1-34 in P. O. Davidson (Ed.) The Behavioral Management of Anxiety,
        Depression, and Pain. New York: Brunner/Mazel.
Melzack, Ronald
1977   "Gate Theory Revisited." Pp. 79-92 in P. L. Leroy (Ed.) Current Concepts
        in the Management of Chronic Pain. New York: Symposia Specialists.
1973   The Puzzle of Pain. New York: Basic Books.
Melzack, Rònald and Stephen G. Dennis
1978   "Neurophysiological Foundations of Pain." Pp. 1-26 in R. Sternbach (Ed.)
        The Psychology of Pain. New York: Raven.
Melzack, Ronald and Patrick D. Wall
1965   "Pain Mechanisms: A New Theory." Science 150: 971-979.
Merleau-Ponty, Maurice
1964   Signs. (Trans. Richard C. McCleary.) Evanston, IL: Northwestern Univer-
        sity Press.
1962   Phenomenology of Perception. London: Routledge & Kegan Paul.
Merskey, Harold and F. G. Spear
1967   Pain: Psychological and Psychiatric Aspects. Baltimore: Williams & Wil-
        kins.
Meyer, Henry J.
1967   "Professionalization and Social Work Today." Pp. 389-400 in Edwin J.
        Thomas (Ed.) Behavioral Science for Social Workers. New York: Mac-
        millan.
Millis, J. S.
1977   "Primary Care: Definition Of and Access To." Nursing Outlook 25: 433-
        435.

Mines, Samuel
  1974   The Conquest of Pain. New York: Grosset & Dunlap.

Monteiro, Lois
  1973   "Expense is no Object: Income and Physician Visits Reconsidered." Journal of Health and Social Behavior 14: 99-115.

Morris, Monica B.
  1977   An Excursion into Creative Sociology. New York: Columbia University Press.

Muktananda, Swami
  1976   Siddha Guru. (Trans. Shankar.) Oakland, CA: S.Y.D.A. Foundation.
  1974   Satsang with Baba. (Trans. UMA Berlinger.) Oakland, CA: S.Y.D.A. Foundation.

National Center for Health Statistics
  1980   Health Resource Statistics. Washington, DC: Department of Health, Education and Welfare.

Neal, Helen
  1978   The Politics of Pain. New York: McGraw-Hill.

Nudelman, Arthur E.
  1976   "The Maintenance of Christian Science in Scientific Society." Pp. 42-60 in Roy Wallis and Peter Morley (Eds.) Marginal Medicine. New York: Macmillan.

Pace, J. Blair
  1976   Pain: A Personal Experience. Chicago: Nelson-Hall.

Parsons, Talcott
  1975   "The Sick Role and the Role of the Physician Reconsidered." Milbank Memorial Fund Quarterly (Summer): 257-277.

Parsons, Talcott
  1951   The Social System. New York: Macmillan.

Pellegrino, Edmund D.
  1977   "The Allied Health Professions: The Problems and Potentials of Maturity." Journal of Allied Health 6: 25-33.

Petrie, A.
  1967   Individuality in Pain and Suffering. Chicago: University of Chicago Press.

Pilling, L. F., T. L. Brannick, and W. M. Swenson
  1967   "Psychologic Characteristics of Psychiatric Patients Having Pain as a Presenting Symptom." Canadian Medical Association Journal 97: 387-394.

Pinkerton, Susan S., Howard Hughes, and W. W. Wenrich
  1982   Behavioral Medicine: Clinical Applications. New York: John Wiley.

Polit, Denise and Bernadette Hunger
  1978   Nursing Research. New York: Lippincott.

Psathas, George (Ed.)
  1973   Phenomenological Sociology. New York: John Wiley.

Reed, Louis S.
  1932   The Healing Cults. Chicago: University of Chicago Press.

Resnick, Edward J.
  1977   "The Pain Center Concept." Pp. 63-68 in Pierre L. LeRoy (Ed.) Current Concepts in the Management of Chronic Pain. New York: Symposia Specialists.

Ricoeur, Paul
  1977   The Rule of Metaphor. (Trans. Robert Czerny.) Toronto: University of Toronto Press.

Ritzer, George
  1975   Sociology: A Multiple Paradigm Science. Boston: Allyn & Bacon.

Roche, Maurice
  1973   Phenomenology, Language and the Social Sciences. London: Routledge & Kegan Paul.

Rootman, Irving and Donald Mills
  1974   "Professional Behavior of American and Canadian Chiropractors." Journal of Health and Social Behavior 15: 3-12.

Rosenberg, Morris
  1957   Occupations and Values. New York: Macmillan.

Rosengren, W. and M. Lefton
  1969   Hospitals and Patients. New York: Abbingdon.

Rosenstock, I. M.
  1960   "What Research in Motivation Suggests for Public Health." American Journal of Public Health 50: 295-302.

Roth, Julius A.
  1963   Timetables. Indianapolis: Bobbs-Merrill.

Sartre, Jean-Paul
  1956   Being and Nothingness. (Trans. Hazel E. Barnes.) New York: Philosophical Library.

Satin, Mark
  1978   New Age Politics. Vancouver: Whitecap Books.

Sauerbruch, Ferdinand and Hans, Wenke
  1963   Pain: Its Meaning and Significance. (Trans. Edward Fitzgerald.) London: Allen & Unwin.

Schofield, William
  1975   "The Psychologist as a Health Care Professional." Intellect Magazine (January): 255-258.

Shanas, Ethel
  1962   The Health of Older People. Cambridge, MA: Harvard University Press.

Scheff, Thomas J.
  1966   Being Mentally Ill: A Sociological Theory. Chicago: Aldine.

Schmitt, Madeline H.
  1978   "The Utilization of Chiropractors." Sociological Symposium 22: 55-74.

Schultz, Alfred
  1970   On Phenomenology and Social Relations (Ed. Helmut R. Wagner.) Chicago: University of Chicago Press.

1964   Collected Papers, Vol. II, Studies in Social Theory. (Arvid Brodersen, Ed.) The Hague: Martinus Nijhoff.

Sergeant, Richard
1969   The Spectrum of Pain. London: Rupert Hart-Davis.

Shealy, C. Norman
1974a   "The Pain Patient." American Family Physician 9: 130-137.
1974b   "Transcutaneous Electrical Stimulation of Control of Pain." Clinical Neurosurgery 21: 269.

Shealy, C. Norman and Mary-Charlotte Shealy
1976   "Behavioral Techniques in the Control of Pain: A Case for Health Maintenance vs. Disease Treatment." Pp. 21-33 in Matisyohu Weisenberg and Bernard Tursky (Eds.) Pain: New Perspectives in Therapy and Research. New York: Plenum.

Shryock, Richard Harrison
1960   Medicine and Society in America, 1660-1860. New York: New York University Press.

Siegler, Miriam and Humphrey Osmond
1973   "The 'Sick Role' Revisited." Hasting Center Studies 1: 41-58.

Simmel, M. L.
1956   "On Phantom Limbs." A.M.A. Archives of Neurological Psychiatry 75: 637-648.

Sinclair, David C.
1967   Cutaneous Sensation. London: Oxford University Press.

Skinner, B. F.
1969   Contingencies of Reinforcement: A Theoretical Analysis. New York: Appleton-Century-Crofts.

Skipper, James K.
1978   "Medical Sociology and Chiropractic." Sociological Symposium 22: 1-6.

Smith, Ralph Lee
1969   At Your Own Risk: The Case Against Chiropractic. New York: Trident.

Sobey, Francine (Ed.)
1977   Changing Roles in Social Work Practice. Philadelphia: Temple University Press.

Sovak, Milos
1979   "Physiology of Biofeedback and Acupuncture: Beliefs and Facts." Paper presented at the Salk Lecture Series, the Salk Institute, University of California, San Diego, January 25.

Stein, Leonard I.
1967   "The Doctor-Nurse Game." Archives of General Psychology 16: 699-703.

Sternbach, Richard A. (Ed.)
1978   The Psychology of Pain. New York: Raven.
1974   Pain Patients: Traits and Treatment. New York: Academic.
1968   Pain: A Physiological Analysis. New York: Academic.

Straus, Robert
1957   "The Nature and Status of Medical Sociology." American Sociological Review 22: 200-204.

Strauss, Anselm
1966   "Structure and Ideology of the Nursing Profession." Pp. 60-104 in F. Davis (Ed.) The Nursing Profession. New York: John Wiley.
1959   Mirrors and Masks. Glencoe, IL: Free Press.
Strauss, Anselm L. and Barney G. Glaser
1975   Chronic Illness and the Quality of Life. St. Louis: Mosby.
Suchman, Edward A.
1965a   "Social Patterns of Illness and Medical Care." Journal of Health and Human Behavior 6: 2-16.
1965b   "Stages of Illness and Medical Care." Journal of Health and Human Behavior 6: 114-128.
Szasz, Thomas S.
1961   The Myth of Mental Illness. New York: Harper & Row.
1957   Pain and Pleasure: A Study of Bodily Feelings. New York: Basic Books.
1956   "Malingering: 'Diagnosis' or Social Condemnation." AMA Archives of Neurology and Psychiatry 76: 438-440.
Szasz, Thomas S. and Marc Hollender
1956   "A Contribution to the Philosophy of Medicine: The Basic Models of the Doctor-Patient Relationship." Journal of the American Medical Association 97: 585-588.
Taylor, Lee
1968   Occupational Sociology. New York: Oxford University Press.
Thomas, Edwin J. (Ed.)
1967   Behavioral Science for Social Workers. New York: Macmillan.
Turner, Ralph
1976   "The Real Self: From Institution to Impulse." American Journal of Sociology 81: 989-1016.
Twaddle, Andrew C.
1973   "Illness and Deviance." Social Science and Medicine 7: 751-762.
1969   "Health Decisions and Sick Role Variations: An Explanation." Journal of Health and Social Behavior 10: 105-114.
Twaddle, Andrew C. and Richard M. Hessler
1977   A Sociology of Health. St. Louis: Mosby.
Underwood, John
1978   "An Unfolding Tragedy." Sports Illustrated (August 14): 68-82.
Waitzkin, Howard
1971   "Latent Functions of the Sick Role in Various Institutional Settings." Social Sciences and Medicine 5: 45-75.
Waitzkin, Howard and Barbara Waterman
1974   The Exploitation of Illness in Capitalist Society. New York: Bobbs-Merrill.
Walker, Kenneth
1954   The Story of Medicine. London: Hutchinson.
Wallis, Roy and Peter Morley (Eds.)
1976   Marginal Medicine. New York: Macmillan.

Wardwell, Walter I.
  1978   "Social Factors in the Survival of Chiropractic: A Comparative View."
          Sociological Symposium 22: 6-17.
  1952   "A Marginal Professional Rule: The Chiropractor." Social Forces 30: 339-
          348.
Weil, Andrew
  1972   The Natural Mind. Boston: Houghton Mifflin.
Weinsenberg, Matisyohu and Bernard Tursky (Eds.)
  1976   Pain: New Perspectives in Therapy and Research. New York: Plenum.
White, Herbert and James K. Skipper, Jr.
  1971   "The Chiropractic Physician: A Study of Career Contingencies." Journal
          of Health and Social Behavior 12: 300-312.
Wiener, Carolyn L.
  1975   "Pain Assessment on an Orthopedic Ward." Nursing Outlook 23: 508-516.
Williams, R. W.
  1978   "Microlumbar Disectomy: A Conservative Surgical Approach to the Virgin
          Herniated Lumbar Disc." Spine 3: 175-182.
Wilson, Robert N.
  1970   The Sociology of Health: An Introduction. New York: Random House.
Wittgenstein, Ludwig
  1953   Philosophical Investigations (Trans. G.E.M. Anscombe.) New York: Ox-
          ford University Press.
Wolf, Barbara
  1977   Living With Pain. New York: Seabury.
Wolff, B. Berthold
  1977   "Psychosocial Aspects of the Patient with Chronic Pain." Pp. 45-52 in
          Pierre L. LeRoy (Ed.) Current Concepts in Management of Chronic Pain.
          New York: Symposia.
Wolff, Kurt H. (Ed.)
  1950   The Sociology of Georg Simmel. New York: Macmillan.
Wooden, Allen C.
  1977   "The Development and Use of Electricity in the Treatment of Pain: A Short
          History." Pp. 19-36 in Pierre L. LeRoy (Ed.) Current Concepts in Manage-
          ment of Chronic Pain. New York: Symposia.
Wyatt, Frederick
  1968   "What is Clinical Psychology?" Pp. 222-238 in Alexander Z. Guiora and
          Marvin A. Brandwin (Eds.) Perspectives in Clinical Psychology. Princeton,
          NJ: Van Nostrand.
Wyckoff, Margo G.
  1978   "The Chronic Pain Experience: Case Illustrations." Pp. 155-61 in Neil F.
          Bracht (Ed.) Social Work in Health Care: A Guide to Professional Practice.
          New York: Haworth.
Yinger, J. Milton
  1971   The Scientific Study of Religion. New York: Macmillan.

Zborowski, Mark
   1952   "Cultural Components in Responses to Pain." Journal of Social Issues 8:
         16-30.
   1969   People in Pain. San Francisco: Jossey-Bass.
Zola, Irving K.
   1972   "Medicine as an Institution of Social Control." Sociological Review 20:
         487-504.
   1966   "Culture and Symptoms." American Sociological Review 31: 615-630.
Zurcher, Louis
   1977   The Mutable Self: A Self-Concept for Social Change. Beverly Hills, CA:
         Sage.

About the Author

Joseph A. Kotarba is Assistant Professor of Sociology and Co-Director of the Program in Medical Sociology at the University of Houston. He received his Ph.D. from the University of California at San Diego in 1980 and has published numerous essays on sociological theory, field research methods, deviant behavior, and health and illness behavior. Dr. Kotarba is co-author, with Jack D. Douglas and others, of *Introduction to the Sociologies of Everyday Life* (1980) and co-editor, with Andrea Fontana, of *The Existential Self and Society* (forthcoming). He is currently studying the social organization of aerospace medicine and professionalization among athletic trainers.